Help! I'm Losing My Hearing

What Do I Do Now?

A Basic Guide to Hearing Loss (and Other Ear Problems)

Second Edition

Neil G. Bauman, Ph.D.

Integrity First Publications

Lynden, WA

http://IntegrityFirstPublications.com

Help! I'm Losing My Hearing What Do I Do Now?

A Basic Guide to Hearing Loss (and Other Ear Problems)

Second Edition

Another **Integrity First** book in the series:

Everything You Wanted to Know About Your Hearing Loss But Were Afraid to Ask
(Because You Knew You Wouldn't Hear the Answers Anyway!)

ISBN 978-1-935939-11-5

Integrity First Publications
1013 Ridgeway Drive,
Lynden, WA 98264-1057
Phone: (360) 778-1266
FAX: (360) 389-5226
Email: info@IntegrityFirstPublications.com
Website: http://IntegrityFirstPublications.com

Printed in the United States of America

Warning—Disclaimer

This book is for your education and reference. It is neither a medical manual nor a guide to self-treatment for medical problems. Do not construe this book as giving personal medical advice or instruction. The author is not a medical doctor and neither prescribes treatment nor treats medical problems and does not intend that you attempt to do so either. If you suspect that you have a medical problem related to your ears, seek competent professional medical help. Use the information in this book to help you make informed decisions, not as a substitute for any treatment that your doctor may have prescribed for you.

The information and opinions expressed in this book are the result of careful research. They are believed to be accurate and sound, based on the best judgment available to the author. If you fail to consult appropriate health professionals, you assume the risk of any injuries. Neither Integrity First Publications, the Center for Hearing Loss Help, nor the author assumes any responsibility for damages or losses incurred as a result of using the information in this book, nor for any errors or omissions. It is the responsibility of each reader to exercise good judgment in using any information contained in this book.

Contents

About the Author

Neil G. Bauman, Ph.D., (Dr. Neil), is the executive director of the Center for Hearing Loss Help. He is a hearing loss coping skills specialist, researcher, author and speaker on issues pertaining to hearing loss. No stranger to hearing loss himself, he has lived with a life-long severe hereditary hearing loss.

Dr. Neil did not let his hearing loss stop him from achieving what he wanted to do. He earned several degrees in fields ranging from forestry to ancient astronomy (Ph. D.) and theology (Th. D.) in addition to his extensive studies in fields related to hearing loss.

His mission is helping hard of hearing people understand and successfully cope with their hearing losses and other ear conditions. To this end, he provides education, support and counsel to hard of hearing people through personal contact, as well as through his books, articles, presentations and seminars.

Dr. Neil is the author of eleven books and more than 1,000 articles on hearing-loss related topics. (See the back of this book for a list of his books.) In addition, he is a dynamic speaker. His presentations are in demand throughout the USA and Canada.

You can reach him at:

Neil Bauman, Ph.D.
Center for Hearing Loss Help
1013 Ridgeway Drive
Lynden, WA 98264-1057
Phone: (360) 778-1266
FAX: (260) 389-5226
Email: neil@hearinglosshelp.com
Web site: http://hearinglosshelp.com

Preface

Losing your hearing can flip your world upside down and leave you wondering how you will ever fit into the hearing world again.

You feel so alone. You feel like no one understands what you are going through. The more sudden your hearing loss, the greater your shock. Fearful thoughts tumble through your mind. Will I lose my job? How will I care for my kids if I can't hear them? Can hard of hearing people communicate on the phone? Will I still be able to drive?

If you are like most hard of hearing people, you don't have a clue where to go to get the information and support you so desperately need at this point. You wonder, "What do I do now? Where do I go for help?"

I want to assure you that there **is** help and support for you. Take a deep breath and relax. This short book will guide you step-by-step through what you need to know in order to live a happy and successful life in spite of your hearing loss.

This book is not filled with ivory-tower theory, but is packed with down-to-earth, practical help, written by a hard of hearing person who has already traveled this same road you are now traveling, and knows all the potholes and bends in this road. This is help you can trust.

My desire is that as you put into practice the information contained in this book, you, too, will lead a rewarding and fulfilling life in spite of your hearing loss.

I know what it is like to be hard of hearing in a hearing world. I have spent a lifetime traveling this hard of hearing road. Come! Walk with me. I'll guide you safely.

Neil Bauman
Lynden, WA

Part I: Hearing Loss—The Basics

Chapter 1

You and Your Ears

Your ears are a vital connection to the world around you. As you lose your hearing, you begin to feel cut off from the hearing world. Because communication is now so difficult, you typically begin to withdraw from your family and friends. Helen Keller once remarked that hearing loss is even worse than blindness because blindness only cuts you off from things, whereas hearing loss cuts you off from people.[1]

There are a number of things you can do to help yourself successfully cope with a hearing loss. The first step is to learn about your ears—how they work and what can go wrong with them.

How Your Ears Work

God made your ears incredibly complex. Thus, in order to keep things easy to understand, here is a greatly simplified explanation of how your ears work.

Your ears are divided into three parts: outer ear, middle ear and inner ear.[2] The outer ear is the part you see. It collects sound waves and funnels them into your ear canal. Your eardrum (tympanic membrane) lies at the end of your ear canal, and is the dividing line between your outer and middle ears.

Your middle ear consists of three tiny bones commonly called the hammer (malleus), anvil (incus) and stirrup (stapes)—all contained in an air-filled cavity about the size of a large pea. A Eustachian tube connects each of your middle ears to the back of your throat.

Sound waves cause your eardrum to vibrate. Your eardrum vibrates the hammer, which is attached to it by tiny ligaments. When the hammer vibrates, it in turn stimulates the anvil, which passes the vibrations on to the stirrup. The footplate of your stirrup raps on the oval window of the fluid-filled cochlea (KOKE-lee-ah), thus transmitting these vibrations to your inner ear (Fig. 1).

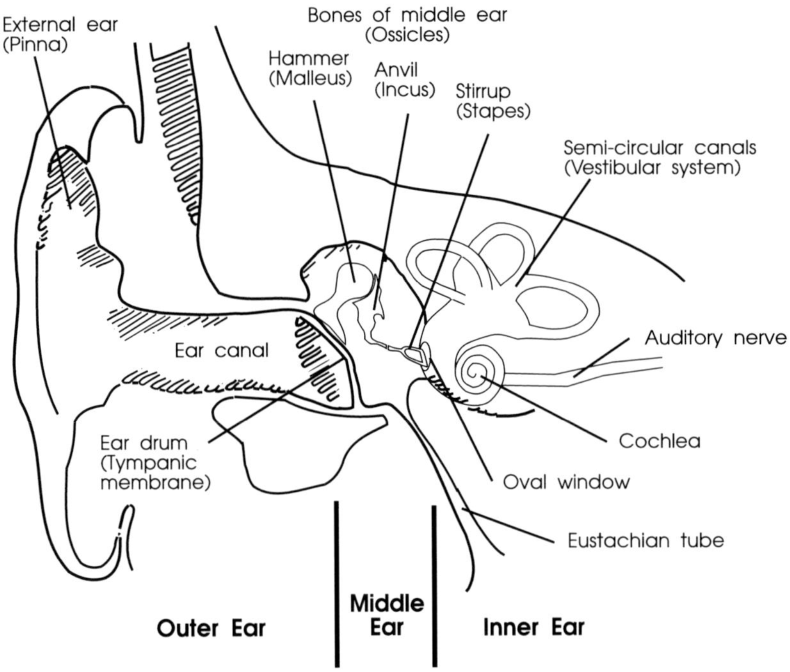

Fig. 1. Cross section of the ear showing the outer, middle and inner ear.

Your inner ear consists of three basic parts—the hearing system (cochlea), the balance or vestibular (ves-TIB-you-lar) system, and the auditory and vestibular nerves. The cochlea looks much like a snail shell and is filled with fluid. When the stirrup vibrates the oval window located at the base of the cochlea, it causes a pressure-wave action in the fluid. This, in turn, stimulates the hair cells in the cochlea. These hair cells then generate nerve impulses, and send them through the auditory nerve to your brain. Your brain decodes these impulses, and you hear it as sound.

Hearing loss can occur anywhere along this path. For example, wax may build up in your ear canal and prevent sound from reaching your eardrum.

You may have an ear infection that "clogs up" your middle ear so the tiny bones don't vibrate freely, or you may have other medical conditions in your middle ear that cause similar hearing loss.

Inner ear hearing losses typically occur when some of the hair cells die, and thus no longer transmit sound signals to your brain. Common causes of inner ear hearing losses include such things as the side effects of drugs; ear damage caused by loud sounds; viruses; and genetic disorders.

How Common Is Hearing Loss?

Hearing loss is much more common than you might suspect. If you are now hard of hearing, you certainly are not alone. In fact, on the average, every fourth person you meet has a significant hearing loss,[3,4] yet you never would suspect this because hearing loss is invisible.

According to statistics compiled by the Department of Health and Human Services, there are now more than 34.7 million Americans who **admit** to having some degree of hearing loss.[5] Millions more are still in denial. In fact, according to the latest information, approximately 83 million Americans have some degree of hearing loss.[4]

As you get older, the incidence of hearing loss increases. According to a March 2001 report by the Centers for Disease Control and Prevention (CDC), at least 25% of the population over 70 years of age have a significant hearing loss. This jumps to more than 50% for those 85 years old and older.[6]

Newer statistics reveal that these figures are much too low. A study done in 2010 reveals that 63.1% of the American population 70 years of age and older have a significant hearing loss.[7]

Incidentally, hearing loss is more common in men than in women of the same age.[8] Hearing loss is also twice as common in white people as it is in black people in America for some as yet unknown reason.[9]

Unfortunately, few people with hearing loss do anything about their hearing losses. For example, the above CDC report reveals that 98.6% of the people with visual problems see a doctor, and subsequently 93% are fitted with glasses. In sharp contrast, only 76.4% of people with hearing problems have seen a doctor, and only a paltry 34% are fitted with hearing aids.[10] How sad that so few hard of hearing people put forth the effort to enjoy rich and fulfilling lives in spite of their hearing losses.

Right now, decide that you will **not** be one of those who do nothing about their hearing losses. Instead, determine that you will do whatever it takes in order to successfully live with your hearing loss. You are already off to a good start since you are reading this book.

Chapter 1 Endnotes

1 Frequently Asked Question: Helen Keller Quotations, 2000.

2 Bauman, 2011e. pp. 10-11.
3 Facts on Hearing Loss, 2003.
4 Bauman, 2008. p. 1.
5 Summary Health Statistics for US. Adults: National Health Interview Survey—1997, 2002. p. 31.
6 Desai, 2001. p. 5.
7 Lin, 2011. p. 1.
8 Desai, 2001. p. 5.
9 Lin, 2011. p. 1.
10 Desai, 2001. p. 6.

Chapter 2

Hearing Loss Is Sneaky! Is It Sneaking Up on You?

Hearing loss is sneaky! It most often sneaks up on you over a period of several years **without** your even being aware of it. Then one day something happens, and you, or your family, begin to realize that maybe you don't hear as well as you used to.

The truth is, hard of hearing people are often the **last** ones to realize they have hearing losses. They are too busy blaming their communication difficulties on others. This was the case with "Harry" and his wife (see text box below).

Spaghetti and Meatballs

"Harry" was concerned that his wife, "Betty," was losing her hearing although Betty heatedly denied it. Exasperated, Harry went to an ear specialist. "Doctor," he said, "What can I do to prove to my wife that she needs to get her hearing attended to?"

The specialist suggested, "Stand some distance behind her and ask her a question. If she doesn't answer, keep moving closer and repeating the question until she answers. Then you will know just how bad her hearing is."

Later, at home, "Harry" saw "Betty" making supper at the kitchen counter. From the living room he called, "Honey, what are we having for dinner?" As he expected, there was no reply.

So he moved closer—into the dining room—and called again, "Honey, what's for dinner?" Still no reply.

(Cont'd. on next page)

Spaghetti and Meatballs (Cont'd.)

He moved still closer, stood in the kitchen doorway, and asked for the third time, "Honey, what's for dinner?" He was shocked when again there was no reply. He hadn't thought her hearing was **that** bad.

Finally, moving up behind her, he asked yet again, "Honey, what's for dinner?"

Turning to face him she answered, "Spaghetti and meat balls—I said—for the **fourth** time!"

You cannot accurately test your own hearing or lack of it. However, if you begin to think you have a hearing loss, you probably do. Likewise, if your spouse or another person who knows you well suggests you are losing your hearing, you probably are.

How to Tell If You Likely Have a Hearing Loss

To discover whether hearing loss has been quietly sneaking up on you or not, check off any of the following situations that apply to you, and/or have your spouse check off those things she thinks apply to you. You may be surprised at the difference between both of your perceptions of just how bad your hearing really is.

- ☐ You don't always hear the phone, alarm clock or doorbell ringing.
- ☐ You have difficulty hearing on the telephone, so you don't use it as much as you used to.
- ☐ You turn the TV, radio or stereo up so loud that others complain, or you turn it off in frustration when you can't understand your favorite program.
- ☐ You frequently misunderstand people, and often ask them to repeat what they said.
- ☐ People may appear puzzled, startled or embarrassed by your answers to their questions.
- ☐ You think many people mumble, or don't speak clearly, when they talk.
- ☐ You tend to avoid groups and strangers because you aren't sure you will be able to hear them.
- ☐ You often miss the punch line of jokes.
- ☐ You are unusually tired or irritable after listening for a long time.
- ☐ Your family and friends seem to avoid talking with you.

- ☐ You strain to hear what others say.
- ☐ You hear other people talking, but you don't understand what they are saying, so you guess a lot.
- ☐ You have trouble following a conversation when two or more people are talking at the same time, so you tune out if there is more than one person talking.
- ☐ You have difficulty understanding people talking if you cannot see their faces.
- ☐ You hear men better than women and children.
- ☐ You constantly follow the speaker with your eyes.
- ☐ You have difficulty understanding speech in noisy places such as restaurants, gyms, crowded malls, in large groups, or at parties.
- ☐ You let your spouse, friend or family member do much of your talking for you.
- ☐ You argue with people and annoy them because you often misunderstand what they say.[1]

How did you do? The more statements you checked off, the more likely you have a hearing loss, whether you are conscious of it or not. Even one checked item is like a red flag warning you to get your hearing checked by an audiologist. Don't be like "Harry".

Chapter 2 Endnotes

1 Bauman, 2011a. pp. 14-15.

Chapter 3

Causes of Hearing Loss

Hearing loss comes from many causes and strikes at any age. For example, Doreen suddenly lost her hearing one day while teaching in school because a blood clot lodged in her neck. In contrast, Delmar's hearing loss snuck up on him so gradually over several years that he didn't even realize that he was losing his hearing until someone pointed out that he wasn't hearing his students' questions.

Bonnie lost her hearing from taking an antibiotic to fight a life-threatening infection. Vera lost her hearing as a girl from the effects of meningitis. Vern slowly lost his hearing from working in a noisy machine shop. Becky lost her hearing at birth when the umbilical cord wrapped around her neck and temporarily cut off the oxygen supply to her brain. Marguerite lost her hearing as she grew older. Andy lost his on the farm working with noisy tractors. Sam lost his from repeated severe middle ear infections as he was growing up. Lynn lost hers before birth when her mother contracted rubella (German measles). Shawn lost his from a brain tumor operation. Jennifer was born with an inherited (genetic) hearing loss.

Noise Exposure

In society today, the most common (and preventable) cause of hearing loss is the cumulative effects of loud noise on our ears. Noise is everywhere. It is hard to get away from it. In your kitchen, you use loud appliances. To clean your house, you use loud vacuum cleaners. In your garage you use loud power tools. Outside, you walk behind loud lawnmowers. On the highway, raucous traffic noise assaults your ears. At sports events the roar of cheering fans is often deafening. Thus, whether at home, at work or at play, you likely expose yourself to ear-damaging sounds.

Every time a loud sound blasts your ears, a few more of the tiny hair cells in your inner ears cease to function properly or die. This can happen in a moment of time if there is a loud blast by your ear, or your hearing can slowly and insidiously disappear over several decades.

One day it hits you that your hearing is not as acute as it once was. You and your doctor likely put it down to the effects of aging, but the truth is that exposing your ears to those loud sounds day after day, week after week, month after month, year after year needlessly robbed you of your precious hearing.

Prescription Drugs and Medications

It comes as a shock to many people when they discover that the very drugs their doctors prescribe for them can damage their ears. There are hundreds of drugs and medications that cause hearing loss and other kinds of ear damage. The fancy word for such drugs is ototoxic (oh-toe-TOX-ik) drugs.

Unfortunately, as people age, they typically take more and more medications. In doing so, they can destroy more and more of their hearing and balance. With many of these drugs, ear damage is not always immediately and readily apparent. You may notice the effects within a few days, or you may not notice anything wrong until months or years later when you realize you have a hearing loss, your ears ring (tinnitus), you have difficulty with your balance or you experience other ear problems.

There are at least 20 factors that can make your ears more susceptible to the ravages of ototoxic drugs. You can learn more about these factors, what you can do to reduce your risk and a number of the many drugs that can damage your ears in the article available at http://hearinglosshelp.com/blog/ototoxicitythe-hidden-menace-part-i-lives-in-upheaval/. Much more information is contained in the book *Ototoxic Drugs Exposed.* (See the back of this book for details on obtaining this helpful book.)

The Effects of Aging (Presbycusis)

As you age, your hearing typically begins to fail. Hearing loss normally begins in the very high frequencies where you seldom notice it. It then works its way down the frequency spectrum to the speech frequencies as the years go by.

Doctors call this kind of hearing loss by the dreadful-sounding name of presbycusis (press-bee-KOO-sis). It is simply hearing loss due to the effects of aging.

As you get older, typically your ears have been exposed to the effects of more and more noise, and to the harmful side effects of more and more drugs. These take their toll on your ears.

Also, your ears react to the health-style choices you have made over your lifetime. For example, if your arteries are becoming clogged due to poor eating or exercise habits, less and less blood is getting through the tiny arteries to your inner ears. The result is that the hair cells become starved for oxygen and do not work as well, and some die. You will notice this as increasing hearing loss.

Chronic tension, stress and worry also cause these tiny blood vessels to constrict, further reducing the amount of oxygen getting to your hair cells. Again, more hearing loss is the result.

As you get older, in addition to the cumulative effects of noise, drugs and life-style on your ears, your ears slowly wear out. For example, the nerve cells in your inner ears and your auditory nerves atrophy. The "electrical energy generator" in your inner ears no longer produces the energy output it once did. Your eardrums become less elastic. The joints between the bones in your middle ears become stiffer. Your brain no longer works as efficiently as it once did. Thus as you age, you have increasing trouble hearing and understanding people.

How fast presbycusis affects your hearing depends on a number of things. In addition to the factors named above, these include how fast your body is aging, your family history and whether you have certain medical conditions such as diabetes, heart disease or high blood pressure.

Hereditary Factors

Sometimes your hearing loss is not caused by external factors, but rather by your own genetic makeup. Some kinds of hereditary hearing losses show up at birth or early childhood. Others don't become apparent until puberty and early adulthood. Still others only appear in middle age or later.

Now that the human genome has been decoded, researchers are beginning to realize that a lot of hearing loss of unknown origin—what doctors call "idiopathic hearing loss"—is really due to various genetic mutations.

Medical Conditions

There are a number of medical conditions that can cause hearing loss. Otosclerosis (oh-toe-sklair-OH-sis) is an inherited condition where the tiny bones in the middle ear calcify and thus no longer move freely, resulting in hearing loss.

Meniere's (min-YARES) Disease (see the back of this book for details on obtaining this helpful book), Autoimmune Inner Ear Disease (AIED) (see the article at http://hearinglosshelp.com/blog/autoimmune-inner-ear-disease-aied-2/), certain viruses and allergies can all affect the inner ear and result in hearing loss.

An acoustic neuroma (ah-KOO-stik new-ROE-mah) is a tumor that slowly grows on the auditory nerve and can eventually result in total hearing loss on the affected side.

Infectious diseases such as measles, mumps or meningitis may result in hearing loss.

Other causes of hearing loss include such things as excess wax in your ear canals, accidents and trauma to your head, infections and high fevers, complications of pregnancy and childbirth, and middle ear infections.

If you want to preserve your precious remaining hearing, here are three things you can do that typically make the most difference. First, always protect your ears from loud noise. Second, watch out for ototoxic drugs damaging your ears. Third, make healthy life-style choices.

Chapter 4

Understanding Hearing Loss

There are two basic kinds of hearing loss. Hearing losses that occur in the **outer** and **middle** ear are called **conductive** losses. Conductive losses can often be fixed by surgery or medical treatment. A middle ear infection is a common example of a conductive loss.

Hearing losses that occur in your **inner** ear are called **sensorineural** (sen-sore-ree-NEW-rul) hearing losses. Sensorineural hearing losses account for about 90% of all the hearing losses in adults.[1]

There are several varieties of sensorineural hearing losses. By far the most common is the typical high frequency hearing loss. With a high frequency loss, you hear low frequency sounds at normal or near normal volumes. This makes it difficult for you to believe that you have a hearing loss, yet at the same time you don't hear higher frequency sounds very well, if you hear them at all. This makes it difficult to understand speech.

Why Hearing Becomes "Hard"

People with sensorineural hearing losses often have trouble understanding speech, even when the volume is at a comfortably loud level. This is why we say a person is **hard** of hearing. If all that happens with hearing loss is that you lose some hearing, then correcting this condition would be easy. You would just need to have people speak louder, or use amplification devices such as hearing aids, public address systems and personal amplifiers.

Unfortunately, when you lose some of your hearing, not only do you lose volume, but also you lose **clarity** of speech. Thus, in a very real sense, understanding what you hear is now difficult. In short, hearing is now "hard."

This happens because typically when you lose some of your hearing, you also lose, to a varying extent, your ability to tell similarly-sounding words apart. Hearing becomes fuzzy and unclear. To you, speech may sound like a lot of gibberish. Hearing aids and other amplification devices often just make sounds louder—but, unfortunately, these speech sounds are often just louder gibberish, not clear speech.

What you really need is both increased volume, especially at the higher frequencies, and increased clarity. In fact, for most hard of hearing people, having increased clarity is even more important than having more volume.

The technical term for this lack of speech clarity, even when the sound is loud enough, is "speech discrimination".

If your speech discrimination was 75%, for example, this would mean that under **ideal** conditions—in a totally quiet room, with the sound set at your most comfortable level, and with the person clearly enunciating each word—you would still misunderstand 1 in every 4 words.

In less than ideal listening conditions, this figure can plummet to 0%. Thus, in noisy situations, you would not understand much speech, no matter how loud it was.

The reason speech discrimination drops with the typical high-frequency hearing loss is because when you have a high frequency loss, you no longer hear high-frequency consonants clearly, if you hear them at all. Yet it is these high-frequency consonants that give speech much of its intelligence. This lets you understand which words are being spoken. In contrast, low frequency sounds give speech most of its volume, so you can hear people talking. Thus, if you can't hear the high-frequency consonants, but still hear the lower-frequency sounds reasonably well, you will hear people talking just fine, but you will have trouble making sense of what they are saying (Fig. 2).

If I'm Hard of Hearing, Why Are Sounds Now Too Loud for Me?

Another thing that may take you by surprise is now that you are hard of hearing, certain louder sounds hurt your ears. You would think that since you have a hearing loss, things would sound quieter, and therefore you could more readily stand louder sounds without discomfort. After all, these sounds wouldn't sound very loud to hard of hearing people, would they?

Not so! As strange as it seems, just the opposite is often true! Many hard of hearing people no longer can tolerate louder sounds—sounds that don't bother people with normal hearing. The technical name for this is recruitment (re-KROOT-ment). Recruitment is another factor that makes being hard of hearing so "hard."

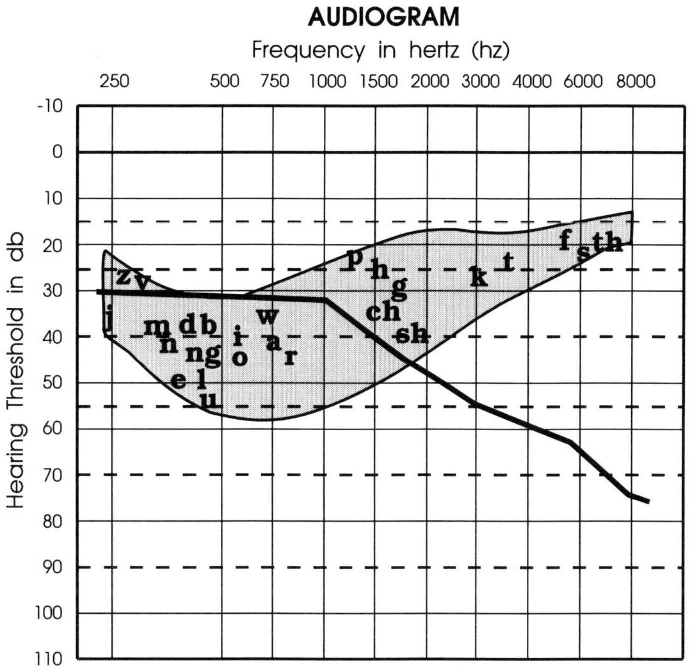

Fig. 2. Audiogram showing the "speech banana" (shaded area), and a typical high frequency hearing loss (dark black line). The low-frequency sounds (below the hearing threshold line) give speech most of its volume, while the high-frequency sounds (above and to the right of the hearing threshold line) give speech most of its intelligence. You can't hear sounds occurring above the hearing threshold line on your audiogram. As a result, in this case, you would hear people talking quite well, but you would have great difficulty understanding what they were saying.

Recruitment

Recruitment is another way of saying that if you have a sensorineural hearing loss, you also have a diminished tolerance to sound to some degree. What this means is that you **perceive** sounds as increasing in volume much faster than does a person with normal hearing. All of a sudden, louder normal sounds become too loud and hurt.

Here is a common example. A person is talking to you. You have trouble hearing him, and ask him to speak up a bit. He complies, and immediately you wince at the loud volume, and tell him to stop shouting! What's going on? He wasn't shouting at all—he just spoke up like you asked him to. This is recruitment in action.

Another common example happens in group settings. Someone tells a joke. At the punch line everyone laughs, but the loud guffaws almost take the top of your head off! This makes hearing in mixed groups extremely difficult for you. If you turn your hearing aids up so you can hear the softer-spoken people, louder sounds hurt! This is also recruitment in action.

The same thing happens when a loud truck drives by, or a dog barks. You wince. You may quickly reach up and turn your hearing aids down, or rip them out of your ears. Again, this is recruitment in action.

The solution to recruitment is not isolating yourself from everyday life or wearing ear plugs. Surprisingly, the answer is wearing properly-fitted hearing aids that have good compression circuitry that is specifically set to control your recruitment. (See Chapter 9.)

Hyperacusis

Hyperacusis (hie-per-ah-KOO-sis) is a condition somewhat similar to recruitment. If you have hyperacusis, you hear normal sounds as far too loud. Unlike recruitment, you can suffer from hyperacusis whether you have a hearing loss or not.

If you have hyperacusis, you have a severely diminished tolerance to normal sounds. Consequently, you perceive normal sounds as unbearably loud, often painful, and sometimes even frightening. It's as if your internal volume control is stuck on high. As a result, just as with recruitment, you may now find that running water, rustling papers, slamming doors, crying babies, barking dogs, silverware clanking, people talking and motor vehicles running can all sound intolerably loud. You may find it difficult to listen to any sounds louder than quiet speech. You also may find you cannot tolerate sudden shifts in volume.

People with hyperacusis are not born that way. Hyperacusis can develop after exposing your ears to loud noise such as loud rock concerts, gunshots, fireworks or anything difficult for a normal ear to tolerate. Head injuries, the side effects of certain drugs, surgery and stress may also trigger hyperacusis.

People with hyperacusis often wear ear plugs so they can get through the day. This is largely counterproductive. One of the most effective treatments for hyperacusis is called Hyperacusis Retraining Therapy (HRT). HRT centers on getting your brain to turn down its internal volume control. In order to do this, an audiologist skilled in HRT fits you with white noise generators. These generators expose your ears to constant sound in order to build up your tolerance to sound again. In addition, you receive counseling on hyperacusis and how to remove the negative emotions you have attached to your hyperacusis. This is a key element in HRT. Treatment may take from six months to two years.

The vast majority of people taking HRT have seen very definite improvement in their tolerance to sound.[2] This makes all the difference between leading an almost normal life, or secluding yourself away from the world. The book, *Hypersensitive to Sound?* (see the back of this book for details on obtaining this helpful book), gives further information on helping you cope with this disorder.

Chapter 4 Endnotes

1 Causes of Hearing Loss in Adults, 2000. p. 1.
2 Bauman, 2011d. p. 30.

Chapter 5

When Your Ears Ring and Other Spooky Sounds

From time to time, many hard of hearing people (and some hearing people too) hear strange sounds that do not exist outside their heads. Hearing these phantom sounds (technically called auditory hallucinations) can be scary and often can cause a lot of anxiety.

Hallucinations—the very word conjures up visions of phantom voices, padded cells and professionals in white coats talking in hushed tones. This is because almost everyone associates hearing phantom sounds with "going crazy" and mental illness such as schizophrenia.

Because of this, few people are brave enough to admit they hear auditory hallucinations. For example, Cheryl says, "I was afraid I was going nuts. I never said one word to anyone about the strange music I was hearing because I didn't want them to think I was crazy."

It's time to dispel the myth that hearing phantom sounds, such as in Cheryl's case, is synonymous with mental illness. While it **is** true that hearing certain phantom sounds (usually voices) **can** indicate mental illness, the vast majority of hard of hearing people hear phantom noises that have nothing whatsoever to do with mental illness. Rather, the phantom sounds they hear are related to their damaged auditory systems.

There are two kinds of auditory hallucinations: psychiatric auditory hallucinations and non-psychiatric auditory hallucinations. People experiencing psychiatric auditory hallucinations generally hear **voices**, animals or inanimate objects talking **to** or **about** them, as opposed to hearing **music** or other impersonal sounds. Such hallucinations are typically signs of mental illness, such as schizophrenia, and should be treated by qualified professionals.

The kind of auditory hallucinations that thousands of hard of hearing people experience include hearing any of the many tinnitus sounds (ringing, clicking, hissing, etc.), or phantom music, singing or "radio voices" (Musical Ear syndrome—MES). (Yes, tinnitus sounds are technically auditory hallucinations, although most people talk about them as though they were in a separate category.)

Tinnitus sounds differ from Musical Ear syndrome sounds in that tinnitus sounds are always simple sounds. In contrast, MES sounds are more complex sounds such as voices, singing and music.

Tinnitus

Tinnitus (pronounced either TIN-ih-tus or tih-NYE-tus—both ways are correct) is the sensation of sound, often a buzzing, ringing or roaring sound in your ears, that comes from inside your head in the absence of any external sound.

When you "hear" tinnitus, your brain actually detects signals somewhere in your auditory system, and you perceive and "hear" them as real. Make no mistake about it, to a person with tinnitus, these tinnitus sounds are just as real as any external sounds.

Tinnitus is not a disease, but reflects something gone wrong in your auditory system. Tinnitus does not cause hearing loss. However, hearing loss and tinnitus can, and often do, go together.

Many people worry about their tinnitus. To them tinnitus is quite threatening. They are sure there must be something dreadfully wrong with their ears or with their brain. They fear the worst. As a result their anxiety level skyrockets.

How Common Is Tinnitus?

Tinnitus is relatively common. At least 17% of people around the world have some degree of tinnitus.[1] The American Tinnitus Association estimates that about 50 million Americans have tinnitus to some degree, while about 12 million have tinnitus severely enough that they seek medical advice. Of these, about 2 million people have tinnitus so bad that they cannot function normally.[2]

Tinnitus gets more common as we age. About 8% of those under 50 have tinnitus all or most of the time. After age 50, about 20% of the population report constant tinnitus while about 33% of elderly people have tinnitus.[3] About two-thirds of hard of hearing people suffer from some degree of tinnitus.[4]

What Tinnitus Sounds Like

Tinnitus comes in a variety of sounds, volumes and patterns. You may perceive its volume as ranging from subtle to shattering! Your tinnitus may be constant, or it may come and go.

At times, tinnitus can be just plain weird. Occasionally, other people may hear your tinnitus (objective tinnitus) as a clicking sound, just like you do. This kind of tinnitus occurs when a muscle in your ear contracts making this clicking sound.

A few people have a type of tinnitus that pulses with every heartbeat (pulsatile tinnitus). This kind of tinnitus can result from an artery too close to your middle ear.

Perhaps the weirdest kind of tinnitus is where people can change their tinnitus by doing ordinary, everyday things such as moving their eyes (gaze-evoked tinnitus), moving their jaw (temporomandibular dysfunction—TMD), turning their head, applying pressure to parts of their bodies or even just by bending over which increases their blood pressure—and for them, their tinnitus.

There are a variety of tinnitus sounds. Many people say their ears are ringing or buzzing. These are just two of the common tinnitus sounds. Your tinnitus may be a ringing, roaring, beating, clicking, banging, buzzing, hissing, humming, chirping, clanging, sizzling, whooshing, rumbling, whistling or dreadful shrieking noise. To some people, tinnitus sounds like rushing water, breaking glass, owls hooting or chain saws running.[5]

You may hear a single tinnitus sound or multiple tinnitus sounds. About half the people with tinnitus only hear one tinnitus sound at a time. The rest hear two or more tinnitus sounds at the same time. One lady used to hear what sounded like a cow bell, a door bell, a tune, a noise like rushing water and a roaring like traffic in a tunnel—all at once.

What Causes Tinnitus?

There are a number of things that can cause or trigger tinnitus.

Hearing Loss

Tinnitus and hearing loss often go together. Here's why. When you experience a hearing loss, your brain no longer hears all the little sounds it used to hear, so it turns up its internal volume control to try to hear something. As a result, it now picks up the internal "noise" in your auditory system. You hear this as tinnitus.

When you treat your hearing loss by wearing hearing aids, getting a cochlear implant or using other forms of amplification, very often your tinnitus fades into the background because now your brain is hearing real sounds again. However, when you take your hearing aids off at night, you will likely experience a resurgence of your tinnitus in the ensuing quiet. One solution is to leave a radio playing on your nightstand to give your brain something real to listen to while you fall asleep.

Exposure to Loud Sounds

Noise exposure is responsible for about 25% of tinnitus cases. The American Tinnitus Association reports that up to 90% of all people with tinnitus have some level of noise-induced hearing loss.[6] If you are around loud sounds, perhaps you've noticed that your ears rang for a while after. That is tinnitus.

Most often, you get mild, temporary tinnitus after exposing your ears to noise, but it may be permanent. The length of time your tinnitus lasts and its severity generally increases each time you expose your ears to loud noise. Finally, if you continue to work, play or live around loud sounds, one day you may end up with permanent (and distressing) tinnitus, not to mention hearing loss.

This does not have to happen. You can protect yourself from noise-induced tinnitus. The choice is yours. All you need to do is avoid loud sounds, or protect your ears from excessive noise by wearing ear protectors.

Prescription Drugs and Medications

Few people realize this, but there are more than 520 prescription and non-prescription drugs that are known to cause tinnitus.[7] Such drugs can either trigger tinnitus in the first place, make your existing tinnitus louder or cause a new tinnitus sound.

Tinnitus resulting from taking medications generally first appears as a continuous high-pitched sound. Often tinnitus precedes or accompanies hearing loss from ototoxic drugs. In fact, tinnitus is the **number one** indicator that an ototoxic drug may be damaging your ears. It also may be the **only** warning you'll ever get. Pay attention to it! If your ears start to ring after you begin taking any drug, you should immediately report this to your doctor. You and your doctor should then decide what to do—whether to reduce the dose, change the medication or stop taking that medication altogether.

Tinnitus arising from taking ototoxic drugs may, or may not, be permanent. The good news is that such tinnitus is often temporary and goes away soon after you stop taking the drug (for example, *Aspirin*). The bad news is that with other drugs it may be severe and permanent (for example, Tobramycin).

Tinnitus may show up very quickly after you begin taking an ototoxic medication, or it may take several days for it to become apparent.

If you want to know whether a given drug may be causing your tinnitus, you can look it up in the book, *Ototoxic Drugs Exposed.* (See the back of this book for details on obtaining this helpful book.) This book contains a comprehensive listing of the many drugs and chemicals that can cause tinnitus.

Certain Foods and Allergies

Specific foods such as red wine, grain-based spirits, cheese and chocolate can trigger, or increase, tinnitus in some people. Other things of which to beware include caffeine, monosodium glutamate (MSG), nicotine, alcohol, marijuana and certain hot spices.

Stress

Uncontrolled anxiety, stress and tension can cause annoying tinnitus or make your existing tinnitus worse. Learning how to deal with the excess stress in your life can eliminate or greatly reduce tinnitus from this cause.

Over-tiredness

If you become over-tired, your tinnitus may become louder, or you may experience a new tinnitus sound. For some people, it is a very loud roaring—almost like a big truck or freight train bearing down on you. This can be frightening. Carolyn relates, "One night I heard a loud roaring sound. It sounded like there was a freight train coming right through our house!" All you need to do is "hit the sack," get some sleep and this tinnitus thankfully quickly disappears.

Ear Conditions

Certain ear conditions may also trigger tinnitus. For example, calcium build-up on the small bones in your middle ears (otosclerosis), pressure problems in the Eustachian tubes connecting your middle ears to your throat, an increase of fluid in your inner ears (Meniere's disease) or any other condition that disturbs the fluid pressure in your inner ears can cause tinnitus. In addition, tinnitus may be caused by tumors on your auditory nerves (acoustic neuroma), changes in the hair cells of your inner ears, poor nerve function due to pressure on them from surrounding tissues, operations on or around your ears, and even such simple things as wax build-up, foreign bodies or swelling in your ear canals.

What Can You Do About Tinnitus?

The impact tinnitus has on a person's life can vary enormously. Obviously there is a major difference between mild or short lasting tinnitus, and loud, severe, constant tinnitus day in and day out. Some people learn to completely ignore their tinnitus so it no longer bothers them. This is called becoming "habituated" to your tinnitus. For others, tinnitus is only a mild irritation. However, for a few, tinnitus is totally debilitating and disrupts their entire life.

You do not have to let tinnitus drive you "buggy". There are a number of ways you can help yourself control your tinnitus. You can protect your ears from loud sounds, avoid tinnitus-producing medications, avoid certain foods, get your allergies under control, reduce your stress, use amplification and get adequate rest. There are many other things you can do. The book, *Take Control of Your Tinnitus—Here's How* (see the back of this book for details on obtaining this helpful book), explains in detail the many thing you can do, and a number of new treatments available to help bring your tinnitus under control.

Musical Ear Syndrome (MES)

"My wife hears music that is not there," Harry writes. "The first song she heard was *Silent Night* sung by a very good choir of mostly men. It came in quite loud. A day later it was the *Vienna Waltz* over and over again so clear it was like being at a musical production."

"I would often lie half awake in the quietness of the early morning and hear a phantom radio," Dick recalls. "A guy would be talking like they did in the 50s. Kind of a monotone voice and all the advertisements like they did back then. It always sounded so real."

"Late at night when I don't have my hearing aids on," Carolyn relates, "I am absolutely sure I hear trucks and bulldozers working right outside our bedroom windows. We are the only ones living on our little country lane. There's no traffic of any kind outside my bedroom windows. My husband swears there are no noises at all."

"I was afraid I was going nuts when I thought I was hearing things in my head after my cochlear implant surgery", Heather remembers. "On the morning after the surgery, I was hearing what sounded like music from a radio. I heard that every day from my surgery until I was hooked up. It almost drove me nuts. Yet I never said one word to anyone about it because I didn't want them to think I was crazy."

What do these people have in common? They are all hard of hearing, and they all hear strange phantom voices, ethereal music or other spooky sounds that no one else hears. Nor are they alone. Thousands of other hard of hearing people "hear" similar phantom sounds, yet they never tell a soul because they are terrified people will think they are crazy. To most people, hearing "voices" that are not there is synonymous with mental illness—not a "glitch" in their central auditory systems.

Because few dare to talk about these kinds of auditory hallucinations, they are thought to occur rarely. In truth, Musical Ear syndrome is not rare at all, but affects significant numbers of hard of hearing people. However, because few people are willing to admit to hearing these phantom sounds, it is difficult to obtain accurate figures. The best estimates suggest that well in excess of 10% of hard of hearing people experience these phantom sounds at one time or another.

Musical Ear Syndrome Symptoms

Musical Ear syndrome (MES), as its name implies, is comprised of a number of symptoms, which, when taken together, form a syndrome. Often there is a group of five symptoms that seem to predispose people to hearing such phantom sounds. These include being elderly, being hard of hearing, not getting adequate auditory stimulation, having tinnitus and being anxious, stressed or depressed.

A person does not have to exhibit all five symptoms in order to have Musical Ear syndrome, but many people with MES exhibit three or more of these symptoms. Be aware that some people have proven to be exceptions to this rule.

Here are some of the more common factors that are believed to cause Musical Ear syndrome.

Elderly

As you get older, your body atrophies. So it should be no surprise that this happens in your brain as well. This atrophy in certain areas of the brains of elderly people is thought to cause musical hallucinations.

Hard of Hearing

Hearing loss is thought to be the most common cause of MES. When you become hard of hearing after having good hearing, your brain feels the loss of auditory input. The auditory parts of your brain remain active, and they may produce their own sounds to make up for the lack of sensory input from your ears.

Lacking Adequate Auditory Stimulation

If you are hard of hearing and live in quiet surroundings, your brain may feel deprived of sound and manufacture its own sounds. Often MES from this cause can be alleviated by wearing hearing aids and/or having a radio, TV or stereo playing in the background.

Musical Ear Syndrome is Not New

Musical Ear syndrome has been around for a long time. For example, composer Robert Schumann heard MES sounds way back in 1854. At night, he heard musical notes and believed that he heard an angelic choir singing to him. He also heard the music of Beethoven and Schubert. He jotted down the music in February, 1854 and called it *Theme* (WoO, 1854). He said he was taking dictation from Schubert's ghost.

Tinnitus

Musical Ear syndrome is often associated with tinnitus. One theory is that the constant tinnitus sounds eventually blend to take on a musical quality. Since your ears cannot generate musical hallucinations themselves, your brain may be converting conventional tinnitus sounds into more organized sounds such as music or singing.

Anxious, Stressed or Depressed

Many times, MES coincides with periods of excessive anxiety, stress or depression in a person's life, especially if the person also has hearing loss, tinnitus and lives in a quiet environment.

Ototoxic Drugs

One lady told how one of her medications "makes music in my deaf ear". There is a comprehensive list of 345 drugs[8] currently known to cause hallucinations in the book *Phantom Voices, Ethereal Music & Other Spooky Sounds.* (See the back of this book for details on obtaining this helpful book.)

Rare Brain Conditions

In rare cases, brain abnormalities (lesions, tumors, infections) can cause MES. The most common causes are strokes, tumors, encephalitis or abscesses. If you do not fit the common profile of being elderly, hard of hearing and living in a quiet environment, it might be wise to have a neurologist check you out to rule out any of these brain conditions.

What Can You Do About Musical Ear Syndrome?

There are a number of things you can do to bring your auditory hallucinations under control. Here are a few of the main ones.

First, learn as much as you can about Musical Ear syndrome. This will reduce your fear and anxiety over the phantom sounds you are hearing. Often this is all it takes for them to fade away. The book, *Phantom Voices, Ethereal Music & Other Spooky Sounds* (see the back of this book for details on obtaining this helpful book) explains in detail what you need to know about Musical Ear syndrome and the steps you can take to reduce or eliminate it.

Second, if you live in quiet surroundings, enrich your environment with sounds. This gives your brain real sounds to listen to so it won't feel the need to generate its own phantom noises. You can do this by wearing properly-fitted hearing aids or noise generators (tinnitus maskers) so your brain will hear more sounds. You can also leave the radio, TV or stereo on, or have people around you to talk to.

Third, if you are taking any drugs or medications that are known to causes hallucinations, changing your medication may be the answer (with your doctor's permission of course). This is especially true if you noticed your hallucinations began shortly after you started taking a new medication.

Fourth, make an effort to reduce any anxiety and stress in your life.

Fifth, don't fixate on your phantom sounds. Instead, concentrate on the loves of your life and you will not notice these phantom sounds as much.

Converse with other people, or listen to talk shows on the radio or TV. This forces you to concentrate on the speaker, and often the unwanted MES sounds fade into the background.

Sixth, accept your MES sounds. Just learning about MES and realizing that you are not alone—that many other people also experience what you hear is reassuring. Once your doctor has determined that you don't have an underlying medical condition that is causing your MES, choose to either ignore them or enjoy them.

If you are hard of hearing and have MES, look on the bright side. Hearing auditory hallucinations isn't all bad. Many people actually find them pleasant. Where else can you hear beautiful music without hearing aids, assistive devices, players, headphones or other paraphernalia?

Chapter 5 Endnotes

1 Jastreboff, 2000. p. 1.
2 Frequently Asked Questions: General Questions About Tinnitus, 2003. p. 1.
3 Dobie, p. 45.
4 McCall, 1991. p. 163.
5 Bauman, 2016a. p. 31.
6 Frequently Asked Questions: General Questions About Tinnitus, 2003. p. 2.
7 Bauman, 2010a. p. 46.
8 Bauman, 2011c. p. 76.

Chapter 6

Hearing Loss and Balance Problems

Many people don't connect their balance problems to their hearing loss. True, you can have hearing loss without any balance problems, and vice versa. However, there are a number of conditions that affect both the hearing part (cochlea) and the balance part (vestibular system) of the inner ear. When this happens you notice hearing loss (and other related ear conditions such as tinnitus, hyperacusis or distorted hearing), plus, at the same time, various balance problems.

Balance problems include conditions such as dizziness, vertigo [VER-tih-goe] (where you have a sensation of spinning), ataxia [ah-TAX-see-ah] (staggering gait as though you were drunk), nystagmus [nye-STAG-muss] (where your eyes jerk sideways), oscillopsia [ah-sih-LOP-see-ah] (bouncing vision), blurred vision, fatigue, nausea, memory problems and visual problems.

At first glance, many of these might seem to be "eye" problems, but actually they are caused by a damaged vestibular system. Few people realize that their eyes and their ears work together through what doctors call the vestibulo-ocular reflex. This reflex controls minute eye movements so you have a stable horizon and thus can read fine print, for example.

When something happens to your balance system so that this reflex no longer works properly, your eyes don't seem to focus or work properly either.

You can learn a lot more about how damage to your balance system can turn your world upside down in Chapter 3 of the book *Ototoxic Drugs Exposed.* (See the back of this book for details on obtaining this helpful book.)

Some Common Causes of Balance Problems

There are a number of things that can cause balance problems. Here are a few of the more common ones.

Viral Attacks

If you have a cold, virus or the flu, sometimes the virus gets into your inner ears. When this happens, it can cause sudden hearing loss and/or all of the many balance disorders listed previously. Commonly you will notice muffled or distorted hearing along with any balance problems.

If you have a cold or virus, or are just getting over one, and ear problems surface, this is a good indication that the virus could be the culprit.

Ototoxic Drugs

There are hundreds of prescription drugs that can cause balance problems. If balance problems surface soon after you begin taking a new drug, or begin after increasing your dose of a drug you have already been taking, suspect that drug. You can find the specific side effects of drugs known to damage your ears in the book *Ototoxic Drugs Exposed.* (See the back of this book for details on obtaining this helpful book.)

Sometimes the effects of ototoxic drugs are temporary and go away soon after you stop taking the drug. Other times, the effects are permanent and continue for the rest of your life. Thus, you want to be careful not to take drugs unnecessarily. Unfortunately, few doctors know, or seem to worry about the ear-damaging side effects of drugs, so you have to be proactive and learn this for yourself.

Meniere's Disease

Meniere's [min-YARES] disease is not a disease as such, but is really a collection of several symptoms (syndrome). Full blown Meniere's disease includes a fluctuating hearing loss, tinnitus, a feeling of fullness, stuffiness or pressure in your ear, and vertigo and/or dizziness.[1]

Typically, Meniere's disease only attacks one ear at a time, but a few people get it in both ears at the same time. Generally, each time you have a Meniere's attack you lose more hearing. Typically, much of this lost hearing returns when the attack is over, but it never returns to its former level. Thus you end up with a progressive step-wise hearing loss.

The most debilitating aspect of Meniere's disease is the violent vertigo. This vertigo can be totally incapacitating—all you can do is lay down and endure it. A milder Meniere's attack may leave you feeling tired, or you may be totally exhausted if it was a severe attack.

You can learn more about Meniere's Disease and what you can do about it in the book *Say Good Bye to Ménière's Disease—Here's How to Make Your World Stop Spinning!* (See the back of this book for details on obtaining this helpful book.)

Benign Paroxysmal Positional Vertigo (BPPV)

Benign Paroxysmal Positional Vertigo results from the "rocks" in your head getting out of place and causing dizziness and vertigo. This can result from something as simple as bending over to pick something up.

Here's what happens. In the balance part of your inner ear is a tiny sac called the utricle. It contains tiny "rocks" (calcium carbonate crystals) called otoconia (oh-toe-KOE-nee-ah). Because they are sensitive to gravity, they help you keep your balance.

However, occasionally some of these "rocks" fall out of the utricle and get into one of your 3 semi-circular canals where they play havoc with your balance, resulting in dizziness, vertigo, lightheadedness, imbalance and nausea. (These same symptoms can result if some "debris" gets into your semi-circular canals. Typically this happens mostly in elderly people.)

Fortunately, the cure is relatively easy. A balance specialist puts you through a series of positions to get these "rocks" to "roll" back into their proper places again. This series of movements is called the Epley Maneuver. You may need a few treatments to get everything back into place again.

Chapter 6 Endnotes

1 Bauman, 2016b. p. 14.

Chapter 7

Broken Ears—Wounded Hearts

Hearing loss isn't just about "broken" ears. Because hearing loss affects your ability to communicate effectively with those around you, it causes a number of emotional "wounds." In fact, the emotional and psychological effects of hearing loss are like an octopus, the tentacles of which wriggle and stretch into every corner of your life. Hearing loss affects how you feel about yourself, and it affects how you react to those in the hearing world around you.

Since communicating is essential to your emotional well-being, how could hearing loss not have a profound social and emotional impact on you? Millions of people go through drastic personality and lifestyle changes simply because they do not know how to successfully cope with their hearing losses. Generally the greater your age at the time of your hearing loss, the greater the emotional adjustment required to hearing loss.

Likewise, the greater the hearing loss, generally the more serious are the resulting emotional and psychological problems. Surprisingly though, some people with mild losses suffer more emotionally than those with profound hearing losses. In fact, emotional problems are just as prevalent among those with mild hearing losses, as they are among people with more severe losses.

Several experts in geriatrics believe that much of the senility of old age is really an emotional reaction to both the breakdown in social communication and the resulting isolation in an older hard of hearing person's ever more silent world.[1]

Emotional and Psychological Effects of Hearing Loss

There is no typical hard of hearing personality. You will react in your own unique way to your hearing loss. Here are some of the many emotional/ psychological effects resulting from hearing loss that you may experience.

Fear

Perhaps the greatest emotion you have when you lose some (or more) of your hearing is fear.

One otologist (Otologists are doctors that specialize only in ears.) wrote on a patient's card, "progressive hearing loss", adding with rare insight "the record might more accurately read, Diagnosis: fear. Fear of failure. Fear of ridicule. Fear of people. Fear of new situations. Fear of chance encounters. Fear of sudden noises. Fear of imagined sounds. Fear of being slighted. Fear of being avoided. Fear of being conspicuous." These are just a **few** of the many fears that may haunt you.

Far too many hard of hearing people refuse to wear hearing aids or ask for accommodations for their hearing losses for fear of calling attention to their hearing problems and its associated stigma.

Passiveness

Fear often paralyzes you, which leads to inaction and passiveness. This is why you may be passive in regards to your hearing needs. As a result, you may be unwilling to do even the simplest things to make communication easier.

For example, Katherine Hepburn, long time friend and companion of Howard Hughes wrote, "Howard Hughes was apparently incapable of saying, 'Please speak up. I'm hard of hearing.'" As a result, he withdrew from society and died a lonely man.

A couple of centuries earlier, famous musician, Ludwig van Beethoven once wrote to his brother, "I was soon compelled to withdraw myself from society to live a life alone". Who compelled him? No one! He did it to himself. Why? He continues, "It is impossible for me to say to people, 'Speak louder for I am hard of hearing.'"

Imagine being so fearful (embarrassed, shamed) that you refuse to even tell people you can't hear them—yet millions of hard of hearing people act this way every day! I know what it is like. Years ago, I was like that.

When you are passive and refuse to do something constructive about your hearing loss, you set up a vicious cycle: isolation, loneliness and bitterness, each producing more isolation, loneliness and bitterness. It doesn't have to be that way, but this is often what happens if you do nothing about your hearing loss.

Stigma

Another major problem you have to contend with is the stigma associated with hearing loss—that of being thought deaf and dumb—with dumb not meaning "mute", but "stupid." Unfortunately, this stigma is still alive today. One study revealed that both the **intelligence** and the **personality** of hard of hearing people is always rated **less** than that of their hearing peers. It revealed that, in general, people associate hearing loss with incompetence, aging, weakness and dumbness.[2] Sadly, some hard of hearing people have bought into this mindset too. They feel that being hard of hearing is somehow shameful and needs to be hidden.

Denial

Since you do not want people to think of you as incompetent and stupid, you may deny you have a hearing loss and put the blame for your communications problems elsewhere.

There are other reasons for denying you have a hearing loss. Liz Wantuch, Ph.D., writes:

> I think we get stuck in denial of hearing loss for so long because we have all kinds of fears of what our hearing loss means or what else we are losing—i.e. ourselves and our world, our job or career, friends, interests we enjoy, etc. All this brings us to feelings of hopelessness, isolation, dependency, depression, anger, etc., and may reactivate feelings about other losses we've experienced previously in our lives. As if this weren't enough, many of us continue to lose more hearing, which only adds to our emotional difficulty.

Another reason you may deny you have a hearing loss is because it is easier for you to deny you have a hearing loss than to accept that the music, parties, theatre, meetings and social occasions you once enjoyed will now always be difficult to enjoy. However, pretending nothing is wrong with your hearing leads to a number of other problems. The most obvious result is your refusal to seek help—if you deny you have a hearing problem, then of course you don't need to seek help for it!

Bluffing

Because you fail to use proper coping skills to overcome your hearing loss, you may resort to a favorite, yet totally wrong, coping strategy—bluffing. Bluffing is simply pretending to hear and understand when you don't have a clue what people are saying to you. Typically this includes such things as nodding and smiling, and saying "uh huh". When you bluff and respond inappropriately, this just confirms in the hearing person's mind that you are indeed dumb and incompetent. That alone is one good reason to determine **never** to bluff.

Embarrassment/Humiliation

You may frequently suffer from embarrassment. You often feel too embarrassed to tell people you can't understand them, and to ask for appropriate accommodations for your hearing loss. You are embarrassed to think you are putting other people out on your behalf. You find it extremely embarrassing to keep asking for something to be repeated. When you only get fragments of a person's speech, assembling this into something meaningful is seldom successful. Thus, you often give totally inappropriate responses. This too is very embarrassing and humiliating! When you feel too embarrassed or humiliated, you often resort to either bluffing again, or quickly leaving the embarrassing situation—sometimes never to return.

Withdrawal

When you no longer understand what others are saying, or feel embarrassed by your inappropriate responses, you do the obvious thing that solves this problem. You withdraw from such situations. Thus, you may stop attending church, theatre, clubs, parties and meetings. In one study, 79% of hard of hearing people avoided going to social events because of problems hearing.[3]

Even when you are physically present, you may sit quietly in the background, not actively participating in group activities. You shut yourself off from the partially-heard conversations, barely-heard laughter, and difficult speech situations by shutting out the world around you and retreating inwardly.

Since hearing loss is invisible, it frequently goes unnoticed by hearing people. As a result, if you just sit quietly and understand little of group conversation, you may be considered dull, dim-witted, antisocial or even a snob to be ignored, again reinforcing the stigma attached to being hard of hearing.

You may choose not to actively participate more than necessary in social activities. As many as 52% of hard of hearing people withdraw and choose to spend their leisure time in solitary pursuits so they don't have to strain to hear or put themselves in embarrassing situations.[4]

Loneliness

When society doesn't make provision for your special hearing needs, you withdraw from those social activities. This leads to loneliness. Loneliness is one of the more damaging effects of hearing loss. In one study, 34% of hard of hearing people felt cut off and lonely because of their hearing loss.[5] Even when surrounded by people, you may feel absolutely cut off and desperately lonely. As one hard of hearing person said, "I am more lonely when I am surrounded by people than when I am by myself."

Depression/Sadness

Withdrawing from society leads to loneliness, which, in turn, often leads to depression and sadness. In one study of hard of hearing people, 60% were often or always depressed because of their hearing losses.[6] Enormous numbers of hard of hearing people feel depressed when they discover they don't fit in any more or are losing control of their lives. Also, chronic fatigue from trying to cope in a hearing world can leave you open to depression.

Personality Changes

Often, hearing loss exaggerates any natural tendencies you have toward introversion or extroversion. When you can't hear in social situations, you may just sit back and become even more passive and introverted and say nothing. Others may perceive your lack of assertiveness as a lack of interest, low intelligence or poor social skills rather than what it really is—trouble hearing.

On the other hand you may try to do all the talking and dominate any conversation you participate in (extroversion), instead of saying nothing. This way you don't have to strain to hear what others are saying since you are doing all the talking. This usually results in people avoiding you in the future, which compounds your feelings of loneliness.

Family Breakdown

Problems conversing, compounded by withdrawal and depression put a severe strain on family and other social relationships. You may feel you are a burden to your family—that others would be happier if you weren't around. In one study, 55% of hard of hearing people felt their partner, friends and families got irritated with them because of their hearing losses.[7] Furthermore, you are more likely than the population in general to experience a loss of intimacy in your relationships. This leads to further family breakdown. In the study mentioned above, 10% of hard of hearing people have either ended a relationship because of hearing loss or were contemplating doing so.[8]

Loss of Confidence/Self-Esteem

When you have to depend on others for your hearing needs, you lose confidence in yourself and in your ability to cope with your hearing loss. As a result, your feelings of self-worth and self-esteem plummet. These feelings are even more pronounced if you are already struggling with other changes such as retirement, reduction of income or declining health.

Fatigue/Exhaustion

For you, listening is no longer a passive activity. When you are hard of hearing, it takes a lot of mental effort to try to figure out what is being said. The result is often chronic fatigue. Thus, you may avoid many social events as the strain of trying to hear is just too tiring.

Stress/Tension

You always have to be on the alert, or you may miss important things. For example, you can't relax while waiting for your appointments. You have to be alert and constantly watch to see if your name is being called. Thus you are in a constant state of tension and stress.

Anger, Bitterness & Resentment

You may feel angry or bitter at the hearing community, and resent them for not trying harder to accept you and include you in their conversations. You may also be angry and resent having a hearing loss in the first place.

Impatience & Irritability

You may feel impatient and irritable with hearing people when they won't follow even the basic tenets of good communication. You think things like, "Why can't people take the time to face me and speak slowly and clearly?"

and, "Why do people insist on speaking with food in their mouths or talk with their hands in front of their faces?"

Despondence/Self-Pity

You may become despondent when you perceive there is no hope or help for your hearing loss. This may give way to self-pity when you think, "My condition is so far beyond hope, it's not even worth trying anymore".

Anxiety

You may feel distressed, insecure and anxious about everyday situations. You worry that you won't hear if anything goes wrong. You are anxious about being in new situations and worry whether you will be able to hear and cope, or if you will once again appear stupid for not understanding something.

Frustration

You are often frustrated at not being able to hear, and constantly having to ask people to repeat themselves.

Discouragement

You may feel discouraged when you ask for accommodations for your hearing needs over and over again while hearing people, especially family members, fail to meet these needs time after time.

Grieving for Your Hearing Loss

Hearing loss, like any other loss, is a shock to the emotional system. Thus, you need to find a way to cope with this emotional turmoil and grief. Grieving constitutes a set of behaviors and thoughts by which you work through the natural stages of the grieving process. The following sections detail how you will likely feel as you work through the stages of your grief.

Denial

The news that you have a hearing loss shocks you, so you immediately deny the fact. This lessens the blow and gives your emotional system time to adjust to your hearing loss.

Some people stay in this denial stage for years. It is important to understand that you will not do much, if anything, about your hearing loss until you are emotionally/psychologically ready. This will not happen as long as you are in this stage.

Anger

The second stage is anger. "Why me?" "It just isn't fair!" You may feel robbed, resentful and angry with yourself or anything that caused your hearing loss. You may try to blame others for your loss.

Bargaining

After you quit denying your hearing loss and after your anger subsides, you may try to bargain your way out of your hearing loss—especially if you perceive that your hearing loss is not permanent. This seldom works.

Depression

When the bargaining doesn't work either, you conclude that nothing works. Thus, depression sets in when you finally realize that your hearing loss is real and is never going away. This stage represents giving up the fight. You acknowledge it is futile. During this stage, your grief may seem overwhelming. You may even decide that life isn't worth living since you can't hear, and this makes you sad. During this stage, you will not feel like doing anything to help yourself hear better.

Gradually your depression and sadness will lessen on its own, allowing you to move on to the next stage. Unfortunately, some people stay in the depression stage for a number of years.

Acceptance

Finally, one day you begin to take tiny steps towards the hearing world again. Only now are you ready to take positive steps to deal with your hearing loss. It may take from several months to two years or more to finally come to this stage. Gradually hope begins to return. You begin thinking of ways to cope with your hearing loss. You are open to help and advice now. As you put coping strategies into place, you begin to feel that life is again worth living. You decide, "Even if I can't hear very well, I am now excited about enjoying life again. I want to live life to the fullest!"[9]

The grieving process is a most important step in becoming well-adjusted to your hearing loss. So important, in fact, that you need more than the brief overview given here. You can read a free, yet more detailed article on *Grieving for Your Hearing Loss* at http://hearinglosshelp.com/blog/grieving-for-your-hearing-loss/.

However, an even better choice is to get the book *Grieving for Your Hearing Loss—The Rocky Road from Denial to Acceptance.* (See the back of this book for details on obtaining this helpful book.) This little book has helped many effectively deal with their hearing losses.

The Rest of the Family Needs to Grieve Too

So far, we have just looked at how hearing loss affects you, the hard of hearing person. Unfortunately, it also affects those around you, especially your family. In truth, when hearing loss hits one family member, it affects everyone in the family, not just the person with the hearing loss. Typically, the other family members miss the free and easy (and intimate) conversations they used to have. This saddens and sometimes angers them. Thus, just as for any other kind of loss, they too have to grieve this loss.

Be aware that when parents discover that their child has a hearing loss, it can hit them hard—almost as if their child had died. In fact, this is exactly what they may feel—that the "normal" hearing child they gave birth to has "died," leaving in its place a "deaf" child. Thus, their grief is very real, and they need time to grieve.

Hearing loss in the family can hit children hard too. When sudden severe hearing loss hit the mother in one family, her young daughter had a tough time dealing with it. Her daughter remembers the day her mother was taken to the hospital. She sadly laments:

> Mommy came back a different mommy. I lost my old mommy. This mommy can't hear. I want my old mommy back!

Because she did not have proper support, this little girl regressed. She became a bed wetter, and she began to have temper tantrums. Thus, when hearing loss hits a family, never forget the needs of the children. They need an external support network to help them through their grief. This is because when parents are mired in their own grief, they cannot effectively help their children.

If hearing loss hits a spouse, and both do not grieve this loss of communication, it often causes a great strain in the marriage. In fact, unless both spouses successfully work through the grieving process, many marriages do not survive.

Part of the problem is that since both marriage partners need to grieve, they are not available to support each other. The person with the hearing loss is busy grieving and needs support. However, the person they turn too in their grief—their husband or wife—is also grieving, and thus cannot effectively help them. Therefore, it is **vital** that both the hard of hearing spouse and the hearing spouse **each** have their own separate support networks to help them successfully navigate the grieving process.

This is what Sally and Bill did. Sally writes, “Bill and I couldn't support each other in the beginning. We were weighed down by our sadness and grief. It was like we were sinking because the two of us together were too heavy for our marriage boat. At this point, I turned to my friends, and Bill turned to his. As a result, we stayed together, but we really did have to go outside of our marriage for support.”

We have just looked at some of the emotions you experience as a result of your hearing loss and the importance of working though the grieving process. Now you are ready to live a full and satisfying life in spite of you hearing loss. The rest of this book shows many of the things you can do to make this come true.

Chapter 7 Endnotes

1 Huning, 1992. p. 9.
2 Kochkin, 1991. p. 45.
3 Bruce, 1991. p. 21.
4 Bruce, 1991. p. 21.
5 Bruce, 1991. p. 21.
6 Huning, 1992. p. 2.
7 Huning, 1992. p. 2.
8 Huning, 1992. p. 2.
9 Bauman, 2011a. p. 46.

Part II: Successfully Coping with Hearing Loss

Chapter 8

Getting Your Hearing Checked

If you suspect you have a hearing loss, have your doctor check out your ears (and auditory system) for any medical causes of hearing loss. However, don't expect your doctor to have a "magic pill" that will restore your hearing. This is not realistic, although doctors can do wonders with certain medical conditions. For most cases of hearing loss, doctors cannot do anything to help you. Don't let this discourage you. It is just the reality of most sensorineural hearing losses.

Below are the typical steps you should follow.

Primary Care Physician

The first doctor you should see in the process of getting your hearing loss assessed is your primary care physician (family doctor). Your doctor can perform a basic examination to determine if there are any obvious conditions causing your hearing loss that can be treated.

Your family doctor may discover that excess wax in your ear canals is causing your hearing loss. He may notice that you have a middle ear infection and prescribe treatment. He may even discover that you have an untreated case of diabetes that is resulting in hearing loss.

If your family doctor suspects more complex ear problems, he should immediately refer you to an ear specialist for further evaluation.

Incidentally, don't expect your family doctor to know much at all about hearing loss and related issues. This is just not his area of expertise.

The Ear Specialist

After seeing your family doctor, you would be wise to see an ear specialist to rule out more complex problems that could be causing your hearing loss.

There are two levels of ear specialists. The Ear, Nose and Throat (ENT) doctor, known in the medical world by the tongue-twisting names of otorhinolaryngologist (oh-toe-rine-oh-layr-en-JOL-luh-jist) and otolaryngologist (oh-toe-layr-en-JOL-luh-jist), is a medical doctor who has completed a least five years of specialized training in treating problems associated with the ears (oto), nose (rhino) and throat (larynx).

Unfortunately, many ENT doctors spend most of their time on nose and throat problems, and thus don't know as much about ears and hearing loss as you would expect. Some are excellent, and others seem to miss the obvious.

ENT doctors that take even more training and specialize only in ears are called otologists (oh-TALL-ih-jists) or neurotologists (new-roe-oh-TALL-ih-jists). These doctors are the real ear experts. They are the best doctors to go to for more complex ear problems.

Your ear specialist will ask you about any ear and hearing problems you have experienced. He will examine your ears all over again. In addition, if he suspects "hidden" causes for your hearing loss, he may order specific tests such as CT scans or MRIs of your ear, auditory nerve and brain to rule out conditions such as tumors on your auditory nerves or problems in the auditory parts of your brain. The results of these tests will help him decide if your hearing loss will respond to medication or surgery.

If there is nothing that can be treated medically or surgically, your ear specialist should refer you to an audiologist for a complete hearing evaluation. (Incidentally, many ENTs have audiologists on staff that do this hearing evaluation right there.)

Unfortunately, often your ENT will tell you, "Nothing can be done for your hearing loss. You will just have to learn to live with it." This is just not true. What he really means is, "There is nothing I can do for you." In truth, there are many thing that can be done for hearing loss. It's just that these things are not medical procedures, so doctors can't help you with them.

To find an ear specialist (ENT or otologist) in your area, follow the directions given in the article *Finding the Right Doctor* (http://hearinglosshelp.com/blog/finding-the-right-doctor-for-sudden-hearing-loss-and-other-ear-problems/.)

The Audiologist

Audiologists (awe-dee-ALL-uh-jists) are the health care professionals specifically trained to do complete hearing (audiological) evaluations. Your audiologist can determine the type and degree of your hearing loss and whether or not you can be helped by wearing hearing aids or other forms of amplification. Your audiologist can help you cope with any hearing and balance problems and conditions such as tinnitus. Most audiologists also are hearing aid dispensers. Thus after they evaluate your hearing, they can sell you the hearing aids that will best correct your particular hearing loss. In addition, your audiologist should teach you how to get the most out of your new hearing aids and give you pointers for successfully coping with hearing loss.

The minimum level of education necessary to become an audiologist in the USA is a master's degree in audiology, but by the year 2012, it will be a doctorate in audiology (Au.D.). The letters CCC-A (for Certificate of Clinical Competence in Audiology) follow the names of qualified audiologists. (See Chapter 13—"National Organizations" for information on finding audiologists in your area.)

The Hearing Aid Dispenser/Hearing Instrument Specialist

If your ear specialist or audiologist determines you need hearing aids, your next step is to find a good hearing aid dispenser. A few ear specialists and most audiologists dispense hearing aids as part of the services they provide.

You can also purchase hearing aids from a hearing instrument specialist (hearing aid dealer). Hearing instrument specialists basically just fit and sell hearing aids. They perform limited hearing evaluations. Some possess a great deal of practical experience, whereas others may not have much training or experience.

If you are not getting your hearing aids from an audiologist, check to see that your hearing aid dispenser is a board certified hearing instrument specialist. If he is, you will see the initials BC-HIS after his name. You can call the International Hearing Society (IHS) at 800-521-5247 to find board certified hearing instrument specialists in your area.

No matter who you choose, make sure that you trust them. Ask around and find one that has an excellent reputation. Your hearing instrument specialist should spend time to help you find the right hearing aid for your specific hearing loss, and he should schedule several future visits to "fine tune" your hearing aids so they will work the best they can for you in all kinds of situations. Good hearing aid dispensers will also take the time to teach you how to effectively use and maintain your hearing aids.

Hearing Evaluations

Having your hearing evaluated is painless and nothing of which to be afraid. A complete hearing evaluation is made up of several separate tests. Each test reveals important information about how your ears are functioning. Most of these tests are conducted in a sound-proof room so other sounds will not interfere with the results.

Your audiologist will use an audiometer (ah-dee-AHM-ih-ter) to measure your degree of hearing loss at various speech frequencies. The audiometer produces a series of pure tones ranging in pitch from very low to very high. At each pitch, you will hear a series of tones (beeps) varying from loud to very soft. You listen though earphones—first with one ear, then with the other. You repeat this procedure using a special bone-conduction transducer (vibrator) placed behind each ear in turn. If you hear better with the vibrator than with the earphones, you have a conductive loss in your middle ears. If there is little difference, you have a sensorineural hearing loss in your inner ears.

During the pure-tone test, your audiologist increases and decreases the loudness of each tone to find the level at which you can just barely hear it. The softest level at which you can hear each tone is your pure-tone threshold. These thresholds for each frequency are plotted on a graph called an audiogram. This audiogram graphically portrays your hearing loss. Your **right** ear is

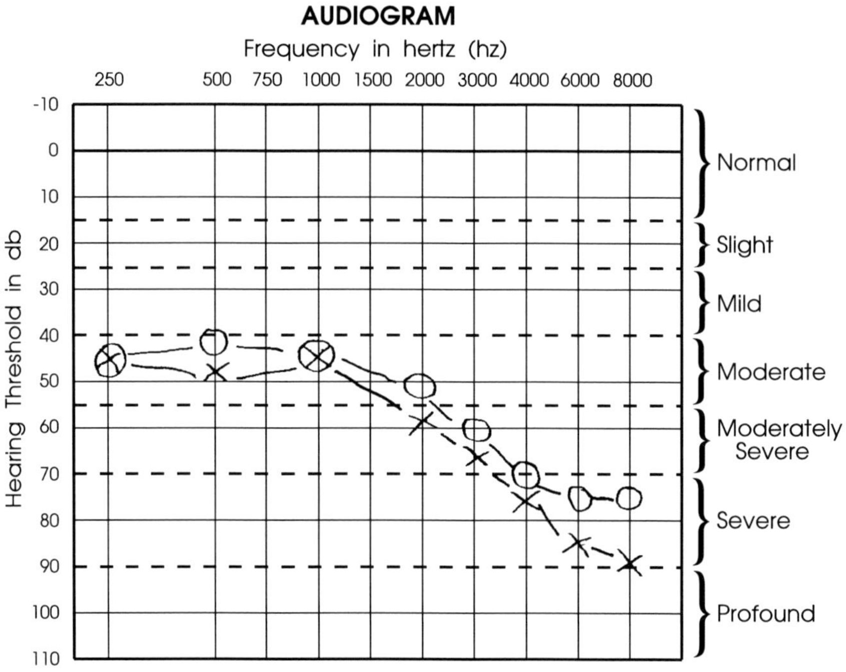

Fig. 3. Audiogram showing the right ear as (red) circles, and the left ear as (blue) X's. This audiogram shows the person has a moderate low-frequency loss increasing to severe in the high frequencies.

shown by **red circles** and your **left** ear by **blue X's** (Fig. 3). The audiogram just shows how well you can hear sounds, but does not reveal how well you understand speech.

Next, your audiologist will determine the softest level you can hear and understand speech by asking you to repeat a series of two-syllable (spondee) words such as baseball, cowboy, railroad, etc. The softest sound level at which you can repeat correctly 50% of these words is called your Speech Reception Threshold (SRT). Your SRT score determines how powerful a hearing aid you will need.

Another test determines your most comfortable listening level (MCL) and the loudness level where sounds become uncomfortably loud (UCL).

Your audiologist will then test your speech discrimination (SD), also called word recognition (WR)—that is, how well you can recognize words (understand speech). For this test, your audiologist sets the volume at your most comfortable listening level. She then says a series of single syllable words that are phonetically-balanced to cover all English sounds. You repeat back what you think you hear. Scores over 90% are excellent. Those under 50% are poor and indicate that you will have significant trouble following a conversation, even when it is loud enough for you to hear.

If your discrimination is poor, hearing aids won't help you a lot. Sure they will make speech louder, but you still may have to speechread and use other coping strategies in order to understand what is spoken.

All of these tests allow your audiologist to determine whether you need and will benefit from wearing hearing aids. They also reveal what type of aids you will need, how powerful they must be and whether you will need hearing aids with special compression circuitry to amplify soft sounds up to your MCL without over amplifying loud sounds above your UCL. This will largely eliminate any recruitment you experience. (Recruitment was covered in Chapter 4.)

Chapter 9

Hearing Better with Amplification

An excellent hearing loss coping strategy is to take advantage of the many different devices that amplify sounds so you can hear better. There are three basic classes of these devices: hearing aids, cochlear implants (CI) and assistive listening devices (ALDs).

Hearing Aids

Hearing aids have come a long way since the cumbersome ear trumpets of yesteryear or even the first transistorized hearing aids of the early 1950s. The array of models, features, types and styles available today is almost mind-boggling.

When Is the Right Time to Get Hearing Aids?

If your doctor or audiologist has just diagnosed you with a significant hearing loss, don't rush out and buy yourself new hearing aids. Read this section first because there is a right and a wrong time to get hearing aids. Here's a typical scenario.

You come home with the shocking diagnosis—you have a hearing loss. The first reaction of your hearing family members is to pressure you into getting hearing aids.

Family members, resist this temptation. This is **not** the right time for a person with hearing loss to get hearing aids. The truth is, multitudes of hearing aids lay abandoned in dresser drawers—unwanted and unused—because family members pressured hard of hearing people into getting hearing aids before they were ready. Let me explain why in relation to the grieving process (see Chapter 7).

Denial: Your wife drags you in to have your hearing tested, and hopefully fitted with hearing aids because she is convinced you are losing your hearing. However, as far as you are concerned, it is a total waste of time because you **know** you still hear perfectly fine, so you don't need hearing aids.

Family member, put yourself in the hard of hearing person's shoes. Would you wear hearing aids if you "knew" your hearing was still okay? Of course not! Thus, if you "force" your spouse to get hearing aids, he will often just give his new hearing aids a cursory trial, take them home, toss them in a dresser drawer, and forget all about them.

Anger: In this stage you are **mad**! When you are mad, you are not thinking rationally. You notice that people aren't speaking up. It's them, not you. You don't need hearing aids! People just need to learn to speak up properly! You think, "Why spend money on hearing aids when your communication problems are not even your fault?"

Bargaining: You have now accepted the fact that you really do have a hearing loss, but you "know" this loss is going to be temporary. You are going to work a deal with the doctors, or maybe even with God Himself, to get your hearing back. Since your hearing loss is going to be temporary, why should you waste good money buying hearing aids?

Depression: When none of the above works, you become depressed. Since you are depressed, you feel that life is no longer worth living, so what difference does it make whether you hear better or not? Thus, you still won't bother with hearing aids.

Acceptance: Finally, however, you begin to realize that you **want** to live life to its fullest in spite of your hearing loss. It is at this point that you are ready to do whatever it takes in order to hear better. Now is the time for you to hurry to your audiologist for your new hearing aids, because **now** you are finally ready, and willing, to wear them.

What Should Hearing Aids Do?

Hearing aids are aids to better hearing. They should do four things for you:

- Make sounds louder so you can hear them.

- Compress sounds to fit your reduced dynamic range (that range of sounds lying bctwccn thc softest sound you can hear and the loudest sound you can stand). This means hearing aids typically need to amplify the softer higher-pitched sounds and limit the louder lower-pitched sounds.

- Filter out as much background noise as possible. This is extremely important as your ears no longer have the ability to separate speech sounds from background noise like the ears of people with normal hearing can. One of the biggest complaints of most hearing aid wearers is that their hearing aids amplify noise instead of filtering it out.

- Provide a way to "connect" to assistive listening devices. As a minimum you want hearing aids with good working t-coils.

Expectations of Hearing Aid Users

You will never be happy with your hearing aids unless you have a realistic expectation of what your hearing aids can do for you. Don't expect the impossible. Your hearing aids will help you hear better—but not perfectly.

Even when wearing hearing aids you will **still** be hard of hearing and will likely need other accommodations for your hearing loss. This is because hearing aids correct your hearing to about "half" of what it was before (as visualized on your audiogram). For example, if you have a profound loss (90 dB), hearing aids may bring your hearing up to perhaps a moderate loss (45 dB), but never up to normal or even a mild loss.

If you are a new hearing aid user, you will quickly realize that wearing hearing aids is not like putting on glasses and having instant vision. Yes, you do get instant amplification, but all this sound can be overpowering at first. You may be shocked at how strange, different, loud or tinny your voice now sounds to you. It takes from 30 days to 3 months for your brain to get used to all the new sounds it is hearing, and to relearn how speech really sounds. Don't expect instant success.

Also, realize that hearing aids work best in quiet situations. As the background noise increases, their effectiveness drops dramatically. Furthermore, hearing aids work best when you are no more than 6 to 10 feet from the speaker. As the distance increases, their effectiveness also decreases.

Because of this, hearing aids alone are not the answer to your hearing problems in noisy situations or when you cannot get close to the speaker. In these situations, you need to combine hearing aids with other assistive technology in order to hear effectively.

One Hearing Aid or Two?

There are a number of benefits from wearing two hearing aids. These benefits are so great that you should **never** just wear one aid unless either you are deaf in one ear or the discrimination in one ear is so poor that it interferes with your understanding speech in your better ear.

With two hearing aids, you will likely understand a lot more of what people say than with one aid alone. Also, with two aids, you will hear sound from both sides of your head. This will give you stereo hearing so you can better locate the direction from which sounds are coming.

Still another benefit is that you will hear better and easier in noise or under difficult listening situations because you can lower the volume so the noise won't be as loud, yet understand more than if you just wear one aid.[1]

Types of Hearing Aids

Until 1987, all hearing aids were analog aids. However, just as with most other electronic devices, hearing aids have gone digital. In between these two basic classes are digitally-programmable analog aids.

Analog aids give the same sound quality as digital aids. Unfortunately, they just have single-channel amplifiers and only one program. However, depending on your particular hearing loss and listening environment, analog aids may be all you need.

Digitally-programmable analog aids have single channel amplifiers, but they may have up to four programs for different listening situations. Also, they may have a remote control to easily switch between these programs.

Today analog hearing aids and digitally-programmable analog aids have basically gone the way of the dodo bird. Your choices now are almost exclusively limited to the many brands of fully-digital hearing aids.

Digital hearing aids process sound digitally—like a computer does. They have multiple-channel amplifiers (between 7 and 16) so amplification can be controlled precisely for each speech frequency in order to fit your unique hearing loss. They also typically have several programs for different listening situations. Digital aids may have other features such as automatic volume controls, noise-canceling microphones, multiple/directional microphones and built-in programs that automatically change the sound output as your listening environment changes. Because of their complexity, digital aids require a lot more "tweaking" to get them adjusted to best fit your ears. Expect to go back to your dispenser a number of times over the first few weeks to get your digital aids readjusted.

Since most hearing aids are programmed to fit your specific hearing needs, ultimately your satisfaction with your hearing aids depends in large part on the programming skills of your hearing aid dispenser. Find one that is willing to take the time to program your aids to your satisfaction, no matter how many visits it takes.

Styles of Hearing Aids

There are about five basic styles of hearing aids. In order, ranging from largest to smallest, they are: body aids, behind the ear (BTE), in the ear (ITE), in the canal (ITC) and completely in the canal (CIC) hearing aids.

In choosing hearing aids, many people look at the cosmetic appeal of hearing aids, rather than their usefulness in helping them hear better. As a result, they choose the smallest aid available because they are embarrassed to have their hearing aids show. This is often because of vanity and/or because of the stigma attached to hearing loss.

Smaller is generally **not** better when it comes to hearing aids. Tiny hearing aids may not have the power you need to hear well, nor do they have room for one important feature that every hearing aid should have—namely telecoils (t-coils). Furthermore, the smaller aids don't have room for multiple microphones, direct audio input connections or integrated FM units. Overall, BTE aids give you the most "bang for your buck".

Get the hearing aids you need, with the features you need, and don't worry about their size or appearance. Remember, an uncorrected hearing loss is much more conspicuous to others than wearing hearing aids.

Be aware that the cost of hearing aids is often directly related to their size. The smaller the size, the more they cost. Furthermore, the smaller hearing aids typically don't last as long as the larger ones. Be prepared to replace your hearing aids every few years. BTE aids may last you from 5 to 7 years and sometimes up to 10 or 12 years. The tiny canal aids typically last 3 years or so and are subject to significantly more breakdowns than the larger models.

If a BTE aid needs repairs, your dispenser can give you a loaner by just switching your earmold to the loaner aid. Your dispenser cannot do this with any of the in-the-ear models so you will be without your aid while it is in for repairs.

Another factor to consider is your manual dexterity. The smaller aids require more fine motor control to insert and adjust them. If you have arthritis in your fingers, you may have a lot of trouble putting them in and getting them out again. Also consider your vision. The tiny aids are easy to lose and harder to find when you do misplace them.

Features of Hearing Aids

There are a number of features that you may want to have on your hearing aids. The one feature that **all** hearing aids should have are telecoils (sometimes referred to as: t-coils, t-switch, telephone coils, audio-coils) because they are so useful in difficult listening situations. It's just plain stupid to buy hearing aids without good t-coils installed and programmed properly to be at the same volume as the microphone. Unfortunately, many dispensers don't even tell you this option exists.

The reason telecoils are so important is that they provide a way for you to "connect" your hearing aids to various assistive listening systems. For example, you can use your t-coils when you are on the phone, or when you are in a meeting that has a loop system in place. All you have to do is switch your hearing aids to their t-coil program and you will clearly hear the person speaking—just as though he was talking directly into your ears. At the same time, background noise is greatly reduced. This makes listening a pleasure instead of a strain.

In addition, with hearing aids equipped with t-coils, you can couple your hearing aids to various personal listening systems via a neckloop, silhouette or music links/t-links—again gaining the double advantages of loud, clear sound and very little background noise.

It is nice to have your hearing aids programmed such that you can hear via either the hearing aid's microphone alone, t-coils alone or microphone and t-coils combined. This latter combination is useful when you want to hear the speaker via the loop system or other ALDs, yet at the same time, want to be able to hear people talking beside you, or when you are watching the TV via a room loop and yet want to be able to hear the baby cry or the phone or doorbell ring.

The current darling of the hearing aid industry is bluetooth-equipped hearing aids. Since the bluetooth circuitry takes up more space and uses considerable power, so far, bluetooth isn't built into any hearing aids themselves. Instead, bluetooth is built into a remote control you wear around your neck on a lanyard. The remote "talks" to your hearing aids via proprietary near-field magnetic induction (NFMI) technology.

If you have bluetooth-equipped hearing aids, when your cell phone rings, all you have to do is press a button on your remote and talk on your cell phone without ever touching it. Your cell phone can be in your pocket or purse for all the difference it makes. When you have completed your call, you just press the button again to hang up. Is that ever convenient, or what?

If you have a more severe hearing loss, a direct audio input (DAI) jack will prove to be very useful. With DAI equipped hearing aids, you can plug the output of assistive listening devices directly into your hearing aids. This may be necessary if the room you are in has a lot of magnetic interference that gets picked up by your t-coils. This interference generally is a loud buzzing or humming sound. Newer hearing aids often have the DAI jack in the same remote control that contains the bluetooth circuitry. You just plug your computer, iPod, MP3 player, etc. into your remote and hear beautiful clear sound in both ears.

Some hearing aids come with tiny FM receivers integrated into them. Other hearing aids can attach tiny FM receivers to their DAI "boots". This way, you don't have to carry a separate receiver and neckloop or patch-cord with you.

Another great feature of digital hearing aids is having multiple/directional microphones. Some BTE aids have 2 or 3 microphones hooked into a directional array on them. When in the directional mode, these aids cut out much of the sound from around you and focus on the voice of the person you are facing, or you can set them to hear from your left or right side or even just pick up sounds behind you.

Directional microphone arrays can be wonderful in noisy places, especially when coupled with yet another great feature—noise-canceling technology. Noise-canceling microphones also cut out a lot of background sounds and make it easier to hear in noise. If you are bothered by noise when trying to converse, consider hearing aids with both of these specific features.

If your hearing aids are prone to producing feedback (high-pitched squealing or whistling sound) you can't hear, then getting hearing aids with automatic feedback squelching would be a good feature to have so you don't unnecessarily annoy people with these sounds.

Buying Hearing Aids

Make sure your dispenser gives you at least a 30-day trial period. This is the law. Good dispensers will give you a 60-day trial period. During this period, you may have to come in several times to get your hearing aids adjusted. It is important for you to "test drive" your hearing aids and give your brain a chance to adjust before you know whether they really are the right hearing aids for you or not.

Caution: Check before you buy to find out which fees are non-refundable in case you return your hearing aid. Typically you will have to pay for the hearing testing, any custom fit parts and earmolds. If your dispenser charges a "restocking fee" on top of this, go elsewhere. You don't pay a car dealer to test drive a car. Neither should you do that when "test driving" a hearing aid. Many hearing aid dispensers charge between $150.00 and $300.00 per hearing aid if you return them. There are some good ones out there that don't charge you a penny.

Try several makes/models/styles to see which one works best for you.

When you purchase hearing aids, make sure they have enough power so you can operate them at just under half power. This gives you enough reserve so that your hearing aids will still be useful if your hearing continues to drop. Otherwise you may have to buy new hearing aids again very soon.

Hearing aids vary greatly in cost—ranging from around $500 to over $3000 apiece. Unfortunately, their cost is not covered by Medicare. Only a few private insurance plans cover them, or help pay for them.

If you need a hearing aid but cannot afford one, there are resources available to help you—for example, local civic organizations such as the Lions Club and Sertoma International. Also, Hear Now, (http://www.starkeyhearingfoundation.org/hear-now) a non-profit foundation may help you.

Successfully Adapting to Your New Hearing Aids

Adjusting to your new hearing aids takes time. It doesn't happen overnight. Therefore, be patient. In the beginning, wear your hearing aids for an hour or so in a quiet environment. Slowly increase the time and noise level each day as you can tolerate it until you are comfortable wearing your hearing aids all day. If you don't do this, you will likely quickly give up and dump your hearing aids into the nearest dresser drawer.

To learn more about how to successfully wear your new hearing aids, read the article, "Becoming Friends with Your New Hearing Aids" at http://hearinglosshelp.com/blog/becoming-friends-with-your-new-hearing-aids/.

Caring for Your Hearing Aids

Hearing aids are easy to care for. If you treat them properly, they will give you several years of faithful, trouble-free service. There are four chief enemies of hearing aids—moisture, heat, wax and pets.

Moisture

Keep your hearing aids dry. Obviously you need to take them off before you shower or go swimming. Some people forget until they suddenly realize they can hear the sound of water splashing. Oops!

More insidious is the moisture that builds up in your hearing aids just from wearing them in your ears. Your ear canals are hot and moist. This moisture slowly builds up in your hearing aids. Therefore, it is a smart idea to put your hearing aids in a "drying jar" each night to suck the accumulated moisture out of them while you sleep. Better yet, invest in an electric drier/sanitizer such as the Global Dry & Store (http://hearinglosshelp.com/shop/dry-and-store/).

Heat

Excess heat will damage your hearing aids. When you are not wearing them, do not leave them laying where they are exposed to the direct rays of the sun—such as on a window sill or on the dash of your car.

Wax

Wax will build up in the opening at the tip of your hearing aids/earmolds. When wax blocks the opening, you won't hear anything. Some people's ears produce wax much faster than others. It is a good idea to clean the wax from the tip of your hearing aids/earmolds each night when you take them off. This allows the moisture to escape better too.

Pets

Finally, keep your hearing aids out of reach of pets. Pets love them! Your cat will play with them and your dog will chew them up. There are much cheaper playthings you can get for your pets than hearing aids!

When Your Hearing Aids Won't Work

If your hearing aids quit working, or don't work quite right, don't panic. There are four things you can do that will fix probably 95% of all such problems.

First, double check that the battery door is closed properly and that the on-off switch is turned on.

Second, try replacing the battery. Also, if your hearing aids start making strange sounds (beeps, sounds like a motor-boat, etc.) or distorted or weak sounds, likely the battery is dying. Replace the battery and see if this corrects the problem.

Third, check that there is no wax blocking the tip of your hearing aids/ earmolds and/or that there are no obvious drops of moisture in the tubes (for BTE aids).

Fourth, check that you have not inadvertently set your hearing aids to t-coil mode. This cuts out the microphone. Make sure you are running your regular voice program.

"Whistling" hearing aids usually mean your earmolds are not fitting tightly enough. Sometimes the fault is not in the earmolds themselves, but rather because wax has built up in your ear canals thus preventing the earmolds from seating properly. Getting the wax cleaned out of your ear canals solves this problem.

If your ear canals are clean and you still have this problem (BTE aids only), check that the tubes aren't cracked. The clear plastic tubes harden and shrink with time and sometimes crack or break. To prevent this, have your tubes replaced whenever they begin to harden—likely about 2 to 4 times a year. The place you purchased your hearing aids should do this for you for free.

If your hearing aids still whistle, you likely need new, better-fitting earmolds. You may need a different style, different material or molds with smaller or no vents in them.

Cochlear Implants

If your hearing is so bad in both ears that hearing aids no longer significantly help you, maybe it's time for you to consider cochlear implants. Cochlear implants (CIs) are similar to hearing aids in that they help you hear better. Some models even look somewhat like BTE hearing aids. However, that is where the similarity ends.

Cochlear implants are fundamentally different from hearing aids in how they help you hear. Hearing aids amplify sounds so the few remaining hair cells in your cochlea can hear them. In contrast, cochlear implants bypass the whole hearing system in the outer, middle and inner ear, and send specially-coded signals directly into the auditory nerve. Thus, a cochlear implant can work whether you have functioning hair cells or not. During the cochlear implant surgery an electrode array is surgically threaded into your cochlea during a one to three hour operation under general anesthesia. This electrode array directly stimulates the nerve fibers in your ear.

Cochlear implants consist of two parts. The external part—the speech processor—looks much like a BTE hearing aid, but instead of having a tube leading to an earmold in your ear, it has a transmitting coil attached to it by a short wire.

The internal part consists of the electrode array in your cochlea. This electrode array is attached to a implant receptor that is embedded in your skull behind your ear.

In operation, you wear the speech processor like a BTE hearing aid and place the transmitting coil over the implant receptor where it is held in place by a magnet in the implant receptor. The coil transmits the processed sound signals through your skin to the implant receptor.

The external part is not just a microphone and amplifier like in a BTE hearing aid, but also contains a speech processor that converts the audible sounds received by the microphone into specially coded signals that your brain can understand as sound.

When the cochlear implant is "turned on" and programmed for the first time, most people describe speech as sounding much like Donald Duck. However, your brain soon learns to interpret these new signals, and in a few days to a few weeks you will find that voices begin to sound close to normal.

If you are interested in getting a cochlear implant, your first step is to locate a good implant center near you. Your ear specialist or audiologist should be able to help you with this.

If you are otherwise eligible, age is not a barrier to getting a cochlear implant. In fact, people 80 years old and older have received cochlear implants.

Unlike with hearing aids, the cost of cochlear implants, including the surgery and subsequent programming (mapping) is covered by both Medicare and the Veterans Administration, and also by many private insurance carriers.

Most cochlear implant recipients find that they hear much better with a cochlear implant than they ever did with their hearing aids. However, there are no guarantees. You need to talk to your cochlear implant center about what kind of results you might expect in your particular case.

Some people can hear on the phone almost immediately after they are "turned on", while others are never able to understand on the phone. Some people can hear well without seeing the face of the speaker, while others find that by combining what they now hear through their cochlear implant with their speechreading skills, they understand most of what people say.

Studies show that cochlear implants significantly improve the quality of life for the vast majority of cochlear implant recipients. In fact, more than 90% of cochlear implant recipients, knowing what they know now, would undergo this implant procedure again.[2] That is how strongly they feel their cochlear implants have benefited them.

Assistive Technology

Under normal hearing conditions, hard of hearing people wear hearing aids to help them hear better. However, two of the serious limitations of hearing aids are distance from the speaker and background noise. This is where assistive technology comes to the rescue.

There are three major benefits of assistive listening devices (ALDs). First, they bring distant sounds close to your ears. Assistive listening devices actually sound like the person talking is speaking directly into your ears. Besides having good volume, the speech heard via an assistive listening device is often much clearer, so you understand more than you would with hearing aids alone. This is because you now hear more of the high frequency sounds that give speech its intelligence. These sounds fade out with increasing distance, so your hearing aids don't pick them up as the distance increases.

Second, assistive listening devices, when properly used, cut out most background noise since the microphone is so much closer to the speaker's mouth than it is to the surrounding background noise.

Third, assistive listening devices can work with or without hearing aids. If you have telecoils or DAI connections, you can often use your hearing aids with various assistive listening devices. Together they make an awesome team! If you are wearing hearing aids, you connect your assistive listening devices to your hearing aids via neckloops, silhouettes, music links/t-links, or by Direct Audio Input—DAI. If you don't wear hearing aids, just plug earphones/earbuds into your assistive listening device.

Personal Listening Systems

There are three basic types of personal listening systems—Personal Amplifiers (e.g. PockeTalker™, Sound Wizard™, etc.), FM systems and Infrared systems. Personal Amplifiers consist of a small amplifier and a microphone that plugs into the amplifier. You might choose this device when you are in a noisy restaurant and can't hear the person sitting across from you. All you do is clip a microphone on to the person's clothing, plug it into the Personal Amplifier, plug in a neckloop, place it around your neck and turn your hearing aids to the t-coil position. Now you hear your partner talking while the background sound is greatly reduced. You can do the same when riding in a car, especially if you are in the back seat and the person you want to talk to is in the front seat or vice versa.

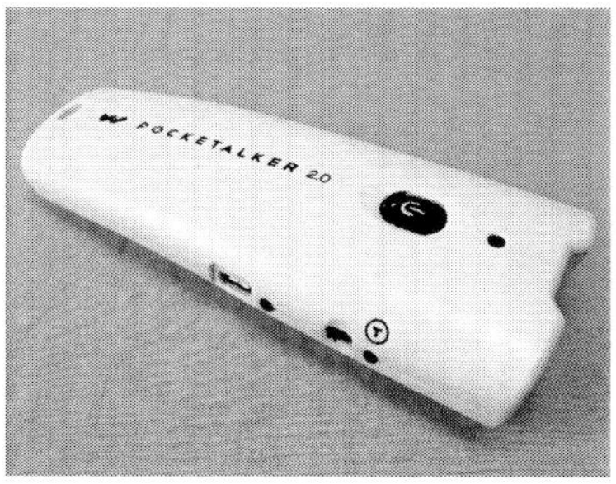

PockeTalker 2.0. Used with a lapel microphone it works wonderfully well in a car or restaurant.

You can learn more about Personal Amplifiers (specifically the PockeTalker™) and how they can greatly benefit you in the article, *Hear In Noise? You Bet You Can!* available at http://hearinglosshelp.com/blog/hear-in-noise-you-bet-you-can-heres-how/.

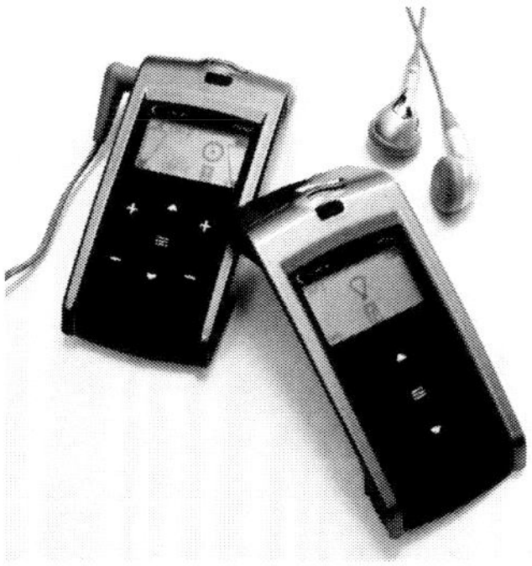
Comfort Contego Personal FM System (Transmitter - right, Receiver - left)

FM systems are for those situations where it is neither possible nor expedient to hook up a wired system between two people. The FM receiver is about the same size as a Personal Amplifier. The person speaking wears a microphone that plugs into the transmitter normally worn on the speaker's belt. You can be up to 150 feet away from the speaker and hear him just as clearly as if he was talking directly into your ears.

Infrared systems are similar to FM systems, but use light waves instead of radio waves to transmit the signal to your receiver. One caution: with Infrared systems, the receiver must be in direct line of sight with the transmitter or it won't work. Neither will Infrared systems work outside in the sunlight. Infrared systems are commonly used in theatres and for watching TV at home.

Phone Systems

If you have trouble hearing on the phone, there are several solutions. If you have t-coil-equipped hearing aids, simply turn on your t-coils and hold the phone up to your ear as you normally would.

Also, you can buy special phones with built-in amplifiers, or you can purchase a small amplifier that goes between the handset and the base of your existing phone. Some special phones even have a jack so you can directly plug in a neckloop or an assistive listening device. If you have hearing aids with direct audio input, you can plug your hearing aids directly into these phones.

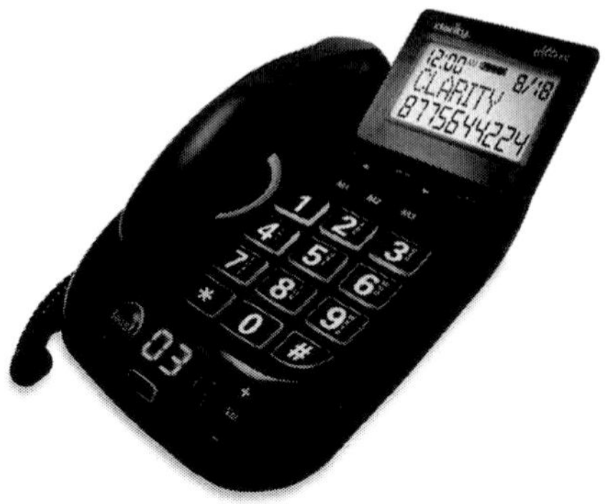

Clarity Alto+ Amplified Corded Phone provides 60 dB of gain so you can hear even if you have a severe hearing loss.

Names and phone numbers can be difficult for hard of hearing people to catch. If you subscribe to caller ID through your phone company, you can instantly can read the name and phone number of the person calling you on your phone's LCD screen. This doesn't help you hear better, but you know to whom you are talking and what their phone number is.

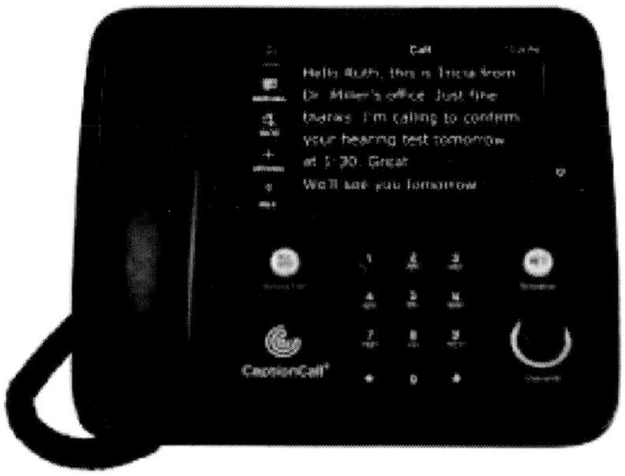
CaptionCall phone not only amplifies the sound, but also displays what the caller says on the screen.

If you still miss much conversation using conventional amplified phones, you may want to try the CaptionCall or CapTel line of phones. These phones, in addition to amplifying the callers voice, also caption what your caller is saying. You can simply read his words on the phone's display.

Television

You can use personal listening devices (Personal Amplifiers, FM systems, Loop Systems, Infrared systems) to help you hear the television better. In addition, most modern TVs now have closed captioning built in. If you don't hear everything, you can read the words on the TV screen. Some people aren't even aware that this technology exists on their TVs so never turn it on. Not all programs are captioned, but each year, more and more are.

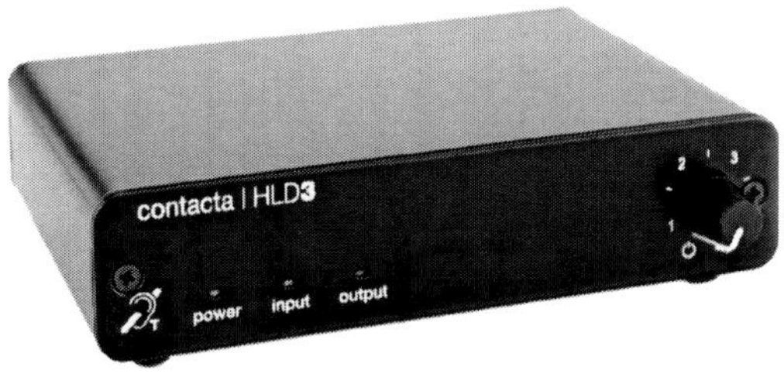

Contacta HLD3 Room Loop Amplifier is ideal for listening to your television via the t-coils in your hearing aids.

Alerting Systems

There are many devices that can make your life easier. For example, you may not hear your doorbell, phone ringing, smoke detector sounding or alarm clock ringing, especially at night when you have taken off your hearing aids.

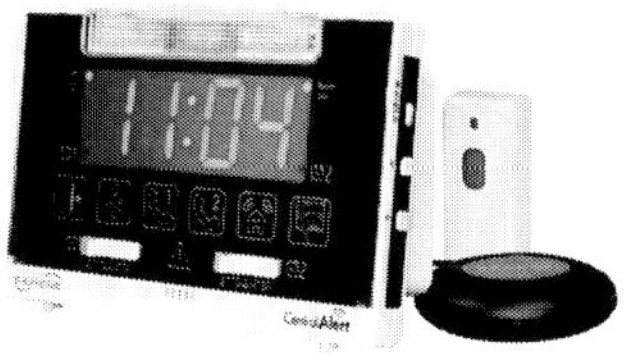

Serene Innovations Central Alert 360 alerting system can alert you to the alarm clock, phone, doorbell, baby crier, smoke detector and other devices.

There are a number of devices available that will both flash a light in your bedroom and shake your bed to alert you. You can have flashing lights in other parts of your house also. Some systems even include a vibrating pager you wear on your belt. It will alert you to the doorbell or phone, etc., even if you are out in your yard or in the basement.

See the "Selected Sources of Assistive Listening Devices" section in Chapter 13 for a list of some reputable vendors of assistive listening devices, or you can see these wonderful devices at http://hearinglosshelp.com/shop/.

Chapter 9 Endnotes

1 Bauman, 2011b. pp. 45-47.
2 Cochlear Implants and Seniors: When Hearing Aids Aren't Enough, 2003.

Chapter 10

Hearing with Your Eyes—The Art of Speechreading

When you lose some of your hearing, you subconsciously begin to rely more on your other senses, especially your eyes. It may come as a surprise to you when you begin to realize that you can now sometimes see what a person is saying. The proper term for this skill is speechreading. It used to be called lipreading.

This name change came about because speechreading is much more than just watching a person's lips. It is the ability to understand speech by using every means possible, including residual hearing, observing the movements of the lips, jaw, tongue and teeth and by interpreting facial expressions, gestures and body language. Good speechreaders have the ability to take what their **eyes see**, what their **ears hear**, what they already **know** about the structure of the **language,** what they **know** about the **subject** being talked about and **put this together** to make a meaningful message.

Most people, whether they realize it or not, are able to speechread to some extent. This is why even people with normal hearing appear to "hear" better when they can see the face of the person speaking, especially if they are in noisy surroundings. This is also why some people put on their eyeglasses in order to "hear" better.

Unlike what you see on the TV, or read in spy thrillers, speechreading is not a perfect art or science. Nobody speechreads that well!

In spite of its limitations, speechreading is one of the major coping skills that every hard of hearing person should learn. The reason speechreading is such an important coping skill is because even with properly-fitted hearing aids, many hard of hearing people still have considerable trouble understanding speech—particularly in noisy situations. Remember, too, that hearing loss and "fuzzy" hearing go hand in hand. Speechreading often lets you figure out which words were really spoken. Also, there are situations where you may not have your hearing aids on such as at the hairdresser or barbershop and someone wants to talk with you.

Speechreading is meant to supplement your residual hearing, not be a substitute for it. To be the most effective, speechreading needs to be combined with amplification (hearing aids, assistive listening devices—see Chapter 9) and other coping strategies (see Chapter 11). This is because some speech sounds are easy to speechread, others are more difficult and a few are impossible as they are formed in the back of the throat.

Fortunately, many of the sounds that are particularly difficult for most hard of hearing people to hear are relatively easy to speechread. Likewise, some of the sounds that are almost impossible to speechread are quite easy to hear. Thus, when you have a hearing loss, speechreading and wearing hearing aids should go together like a hand in a well-fitting glove.

The proper way is to hear what you can, speechread what you can, and let your brain put them both together to give you the whole message.

In truth, understanding speech increases dramatically when you combine amplification and practice other coping strategies at the same time as you are speechreading. Even a tiny bit of hearing makes speechreading much easier than trying to speechread in total silence. For example, one lady found that she could speechread 34% without her hearing aids. With her hearing aids, but not speechreading, she could only get 16% since she has a profound hearing loss. However, combining wearing hearing aids and speechreading, she understood 88%, a very significant improvement![1]

Speechreading Limitations

Before you embark on a speechreading course, you need to have realistic expectations of what speechreading can and cannot do. Speechreading has a number of serious limitations. Here is why speechreading is not an easy skill to pick up and use.

- **Speechreading isn't an exact science.** This is because when we speak English, we move our mouths to produce **distinctive sounds**, **not** to produce **distinctive lip movements**. There is no one-to-one correlation between lip movements and speech sounds.

- **One mouth shape may produce several sounds.** This makes speechreading ambiguous if you cannot hear. Words and syllables that look the same on a person's mouth, but that have different sounds are called homophenes (HOME-oh-feenz). For example in the sentence, "Buy my pie," all three words have identical lip movements. Thus, there is no way to know whether the person really said, "Buy my pie," or "My, my, my," or "Buy, buy, buy." There are numerous homophenes in English. For example, the words "shoot," "shoes," "chews," "juice" and "June" look exactly the same on a person's lips. So do words as different as "queen" and "white; the colors "red," "green" and "grey;" the words "chirp" and "germ" and many, many others.

- **You can only speechread a language that you both know and speak.** This is because in speechreading, you focus on recognizing patterns of words and phrases rather than on just identifying syllables or words. To be successful, you must know all the words being spoken, and they must be in the normal word order. Incidentally, when you know the language, you can often predict the presence of sounds/words you cannot see. When you are speechreading, focus on the overall meaning of the message, not on the specific details of each syllable or word.

- **In order for a sound to be easily speechread, it must be formed on the lips and/or in the front of the mouth.** English is not a particularly easy language to speechread because we form many sounds in the middle or back of our mouths. The best estimates are that only 30 to 40% of English sounds can be speechread.[2] This is why it is generally necessary to hear some sounds. Otherwise, you have to do a lot of educated guessing.

- **You can only speechread people when you can clearly see their faces.** If they turn away or the light is poor, you will miss much or everything.

- **People talk too fast to speechread effectively.** If the person you are trying to speechread is talking at a normal rate, you will likely miss between one quarter and one half of what they say just because your eyes and brain can't keep up with all the rapidly-changing lip shapes. Speechreading skill greatly improves if the person you are speechreading speaks slowly and clearly, and leaves some pauses so your brain can catch up.

- **Some people are very easy to speechread.** However, about 10% of the population move their lips in such a way that it is **absolutely impossible** to speechread even one word they say.[3] Fortunately, most people fall somewhere in between. When you speechread one person well, your family/friends might think that you can do that with anyone. This is just **not** true.

- **Speechreading requires intense concentration.** Speechreaders must follow every lip movement, every facial expression and every gesture in order to try to find meaning in what a person is saying. You cannot relax your eyes for even a split second. A hearing person can look away yet still listen, but you must pay close attention all the time. Furthermore, speechreading is not just about watching speech movements, but it also includes considerable mental effort in making sense from an incompletely received message. As a result, speechreading is very tiring, especially with someone who is hard to speechread in the first place. To overcome this, you should rest both your eyes and brain from time to time. Staring into the distance for a few seconds and letting your mind go blank often does the trick.

Tips for Becoming a Better Speechreader

- You can only listen with your eyes if you have clear vision. Be sure the prescription for your glasses is up to date, and that you are wearing properly-fitted glasses if you need them.

- Be patient. Speechreading can't be learned in a day, or a week, or a month. You will notice that you continue to improve the longer you speechread.

- Optimal conditions for speechreading are when the person speaking is facing the light, you are between three and six feet from the speaker and you are on the same level as the speaker.

- Concentrate on watching the speaker's face, lips and body language when they are speaking. This requires your undivided attention. If you once had good hearing, you are used to getting much information though your ears. Now, you have to give priority to visual clues.

- The one bad habit that absolutely guarantees you will fail at speechreading is **not watching** a person's face **at all times**. The real secret to speechreading is always watching the speaker's face. Stare at them! Never take your eyes off them. Practice, practice, practice. A good speechreader practices speechreading whenever anyone around is speaking.

- Speechread for thought or content rather than trying to understand each individual word. You are really interested in sentences, not individual sounds. Your aim is to understand the basic thoughts people are saying.

- Watch for non-verbal clues. Body language can be a great help in understanding a conversation.

- In order to speechread well, you must know ahead of time what subject people are talking about. Knowing the context is very important. It is also important to keep up to date with news events so you are knowledgeable about likely subjects of conversation. It is ever so much easier to speechread when you are familiar with the topic being discussed.

Speechreading is neither an easy skill to acquire, nor is it anywhere near 100% accurate. However, it is indispensable to multitudes of hard of hearing people who use it every day in order to help them effectively communicate with others. I am one of these. With hard work, perseverance and practice, you can do the same.

Chapter 10 Endnotes

1 Holman, 2002.
2 Staab, 1991. p. 83.
3 Kisor, 1990. p. xv.

Chapter 11

Strategies That Make Talking with Hard of Hearing People Easier

This chapter is aimed at hearing people and what you (hearing people) can do on your part to help us (hard of hearing people) hear better. Remember, communication is a two-way street. **Both** people in the conversation have to do their part.

Hearing people take effortless communication for granted. Hearing for you is easy. This is not true for us. As hard of hearing people, we generally struggle to understand everything we hear.

Listening conditions must be right in order for us to be able to hear and understand you. Unlike you, we can't just "listen harder". We are already giving more than 100% and still miss a lot.

Since we are already doing all we can in order to keep up our end of the conversation, the rest is up to you. We need every bit of help you can give us. In short, we need you to change your normal conversation patterns to fit our needs. By putting the following tips into practice, you will make it possible for us to hear you better. This will make the difference between both of us having a comfortable chat, or experiencing an exercise in futility that leaves both of us frustrated.

Here are some things you (hearing person) can do to greatly improve conversation with us (hard of hearing people). **These things are not optional**. If you do not follow them, chances are we simply will not understand you.

- Get our attention **before** you speak. Either approach us in our line of vision, wave at us or touch us on the shoulder or arm to get our attention, then **wait** until we focus on your face before you begin to speak.

- Face us while you are talking to us. This is **very** important. Notice that I did not say you **should** face us when talking to us. There is no gray area here. If you want to communicate effectively with us, (and save yourself a lot of repetition and aggravation in the process) you **must** look at us. (Of course, this implies, too, that we are also looking at you!)

Andy & His Grandson

Andy's four-year-old grandson, Evan, had been instructed to always look at him when he wanted to talk to him because Andy is now severely hard of hearing. One day as Andy was going out the back door to do some chores on the farm, Evan called out from behind him, "Grandpa, can I come with you?"

"Now, Evan," his mother admonished him, "you know that grandpa can't hear you when you are not looking at him."

"But mommy," protested Evan staring at Andy's rapidly disappearing back, "I **am** looking at him!"

Facing us does two things. First, it makes it possible for us to speechread you. It is almost impossible for us to understand you if we cannot see your lips, facial expressions and gestures. Second, it aims the sound directly at our ears so we can hear you better.

- Get close to us before you begin talking. This is another point that is not optional if we are to hear you. Even just getting a few feet closer can make a tremendous difference. The ideal distance for conversing with us is just 3 to 6 feet. At that distance, our hearing aids will pick up your voice the best, and we will be able to speechread you clearly.

- Don't speak or call to us from another room. We need to see your face in order to speechread. Also, the extra distance distorts your voice (if we even hear you at all).

- Don't mumble. Speak up a bit louder than normal, but **never** shout at us because many of us have recruitment. If we wince or quickly reach up to turn our hearing aids down, you are talking too loudly. Also, shouting distorts both your voice and your lip movements, making it even more difficult for us to understand you. Besides, it often embarrasses us.

- Hold your voice at a steady, comfortable volume. When you let your voice trail off we no longer hear you. Also, **never** lower your voice for emphasis, such as many people do when coming to the punch line of a joke. If you do, we will completely miss the point of your joke.

- Another characteristic of being hard of hearing is that our ears cannot separate speech from other sounds like your ears can. Therefore, cut out as much background noise as possible before you talk to us. It will make it so much easier for us to understand you. As the volume of the background noise goes up, our comprehension drops dramatically. Thus, we generally cannot understand you in the presence of running water, rustling papers, the vacuum cleaner or other noisy household appliances running; other people talking; or while trying to hear you through the noise of the TV, radio or stereo. To you, soothing background music may create the right mood. To us, it is just more obnoxious noise we have to try to hear you through. Also, shut doors and close windows if noise is coming in from outside.

- We need adequate light on your face so we can speechread you. Almost all hard of hearing people speechread to some extent, although many do not even realize they do it.

  The direction from which the light is coming is important. Make sure the light falls on your face and not in our eyes. In practical terms, do not stand in front of a light or window. If you have the light behind you, it will put your face in a shadow. If your face is in the shadow, it will be difficult or impossible for us to speechread you.

  Also, if the light source is behind you, we have to squint to try to get the important visual information we need to understand you. This is decidedly difficult when our eyes are narrowed to tiny slits.

- Use lots of facial expressions and gestures. Be animated. Do whatever is necessary to get your message across. By all means, use meaningful gestures (just avoid extraneous motions which can distract us from what you are saying). Being more animated makes it ever so much easier for us to "catch" what you are saying as compared to just speaking with a "deadpan" expression on your face. At the very least, we will know if what you are saying is funny, or sad, or serious.

- Speak clearly but don't over-enunciate. You don't want to distort your voice or your lips.

- Speak a bit **slower** than usual. There is a very good reason for this. Hard of hearing people normally speechread as well as listen with their ears. People speaking at a normal rate make about 13 to 15 lip movements per second. Unfortunately, our eyes (and brains) are only able to distinguish and process about 8 or 9 lip movements a second.[1] Speaking slowly gives our brains enough time to translate your lip movements into the words you are saying. If you talk too fast, we just fall further and further behind and never do catch what you are saying.

- Speak simply using common English words in complete sentences so we can get the whole thought in its proper context. You make it much more difficult for us to understand you when you use big or uncommon words and/or long involved sentences. Another thing that easily confuses us is when you suddenly return to a previous thought in the middle of a sentence. We aren't sure if we are hearing a garbled message because of our hearing losses, or if you simply interrupted your thoughts in midstream.

- Do not call to us from another room and expect us to understand you. If you are in a different room, somebody has to move! Here is the fair way to do it. If you want to talk to us, it is your responsibility to come to where we are. Don't expect us to come running to you. By the same token, if we want to talk to you (and you are in another room), we will come to you.

- Don't eat or chew gum, or otherwise distort your facial movements when talking to us. If you do, your speech will be difficult for us to understand. All that extra lip flapping and jaw movement confuses us. Just the opposite happens when you try to talk with a cigarette in your mouth—you don't move your lips enough for us to speechread you.

- Keep your head still when you are speaking. Don't bob it around or keep looking around or down. We like it best when you just focus on us.

- Keep your hands away from your face—especially your mouth—when you are talking. Some people just seem to have to wave their hands when they talk. That's okay, just keep them away from your face. Covering your mouth also muffles the sound of your voice.

- Speechreading is considerably harder if you wear a moustache or beard. Full beards and mustaches overhanging the top lip make speechreading impossible. If you regularly talk to hard of hearing people, shave off your beard and moustache. It's that important! This is especially true for bearded men in the health care professions such as doctors, audiologists and ear specialists, and for male teachers and educators at all levels.

- Treat us as intelligent human beings. We are struggling to understand you. In fact, we feel even more frustrated than you do when you are not getting through to us. Always keep in mind that we are "deaf," not "daft!" If you say something, and we don't get it the first time, don't say, "Forget it!" or "Never mind!" or "It wasn't important." or "It doesn't matter." or worse yet, "Pay attention!" If it was important enough for you to say it once, it is important enough for you to repeat until we get it. Accord us the same courtesy you would extend to your hearing friends and repeat it again.

- If we miss something you say, repeat it again (and again if necessary). Sometimes we just cannot seem to get a word or phrase no matter how much you repeat it. If this happens, rephrase it using other words. Often this helps. If we still don't get it, please write down the key words for us.

- Be patient with us when we do not understand you the first time (and you have to repeat it again). Never show your impatience or signs of annoyance. That is one sure way to quickly squelch any further communication between us. We feel bad enough not being able to understand you, without causing you annoyance too.

  Also, be patient with us if we do not get your name right the first time. We find it extremely difficult to speechread names. Because a name has no context to determine what it will be, we do not have any clues to help us. If you have a foreign or unusual name, please write it down. We will never get it otherwise.

- Provide visual clues, especially if changing the subject. It may be as simple as pointing to the next item or object so we know where to look/go next.

- Watch our facial expressions. If we are frowning or looking puzzled, that is a strong indication we have not understood you. Stop and repeat your last point again. You'll just be wasting your breath if you continue on. When we finally get it, we will often nod or smile.

Similarly, if we do not laugh at your jokes, likely we didn't hear the punch line because you lowered your voice a bit for emphasis. When this happens, all you need to do is repeat the punch line without dropping your voice.

- Watch our body language. For example, if you move to talk into our ears and we pull back, don't continue to try. In many cases, we need to see your face to speechread. Also, we may need to get back far enough so our eyes can focus clearly on your face.

  On the other hand, if we are leaning towards you, that is a clue we are straining to hear and you need to speak up, enunciate more clearly and/or move closer to us.

- Speak to our better ear if we hear better in one ear than the other. You can probably tell if we have a better ear because we will likely turn that ear towards you. If you notice that we are leaning to you with our left ear, talk to that ear. Don't try to speak to our other ear. Likely it isn't working. Also, unless it is dark, or we are also blind, never speak directly into our ears. If you do, we can't see your face, so we lose all those vital visual clues we need to help us understand you.

- Converse with us one-to-one as much as possible. This makes a tremendous difference to our understanding you. Even adding just one other person to the conversation often causes our comprehension to drop dramatically. Always remember that our ears cannot separate people's voices like your ears can. That is why in most group situations, we hear people talking, but cannot understand much of what they say. Also, we find it difficult to follow several people at once. By the time we have figured out who is speaking next, we have lost most of what was said. It is much easier for us to understand you face-to-face in a quiet corner of the room than as a member of a small group.

- We need listening breaks if you have been talking for a long time, or if we have been trying to hear you under difficult listening conditions. Speechreading and straining to hear are exhausting. Our eyes get tired as well as our brains, so from time to time give us a chance to rest for a few minutes.

- Ask us what you need to do so we can hear you better. Often one or two of the above points will make all the difference. You may think you need to speak up, but maybe we really need you to speak slower or close the blinds behind you. Don't bother trying to guess. Just ask.[2]

To learn more about how to talk to hard of hearing people, especially in groups, hospitals and under emergency conditions, read *Talking With Hard of Hearing People—Here's How To Do It Right!* (See the back of this book for details on obtaining this helpful book.)

Chapter 11 Endnotes

1 Alpiner, 1987. p. 306.

2 Bauman, 2010b. pp. 9-15.

Chapter 12

If You Don't Advocate for Yourself, Who Will?

One of the most important, yet one of the least understood coping skills you need to learn in order to successfully cope with your hearing loss is learning how to advocate effectively for your own hearing needs. You may find that learning to speak up and advocate for yourself is the most difficult coping skill you need to master. This is because you neither want to impose on others, nor do you want to draw attention to yourself and your hearing loss. Thus, you often just sit and suffer in silence. At the same time, the hearing people around you do not even know anything is wrong.

Unless you assert yourself, hearing people will never know the proper way to communicate with you. Hearing people are not mind-readers. They think, feel and act as hearing people. Thus, they are often unaware of the specific hearing needs you have. If you are going to communicate effectively with hearing people, you need to speak up and let the hearing people know what your specific needs are. This is advocating for yourself.

There are three approaches you can use when advocating for yourself. You can either be passive, aggressive or assertive.

Passive

Enormous numbers of hard of hearing people are passive regarding their hearing needs. Down deep, passive people hope others will guess what they need without their having to say or do anything. The main characteristic of passive people is that they put the needs of others **ahead** of their own needs. Instead of admitting that their needs are equally as important as the needs of others—they choose not to draw attention to themselves. As a result, their needs go unmet. This attitude leads to low self-esteem and resentment towards the hearing world.

Typically, if you are passive, you will withdraw from family and friends, pretend to understand when you don't (bluffing), avoid social situations and ignore others when you can't hear them. This results in your appearing foolish or stupid when you respond inappropriately. In addition, you often feel frustrated and your self-esteem plummets.

Aggressive

Aggressive behavior is the opposite of passive behavior and is equally bad. The main characteristic of aggressive people is that they consider **only** their own needs and ride roughshod over the needs of others. Few hard of hearing people are naturally aggressive. However, some passive hard of hearing people, after holding their anger and resentment in for years, finally explode and exhibit aggressive behavior.

If you are aggressive, you try to shift the blame for your hearing problems to others. It is always someone else's fault you can't hear. You say things like, "If you only would speak up, I could hear you."

You may accuse others of mumbling, deny you have a hearing problem, dominate the conversation so you don't have to try to hear others, and blame others for any resulting communications problems. This aggressive behavior is obnoxious and alienates everyone around you, yet does nothing to correct the underlying communications problems.

Assertive

As a hard of hearing people, you need to be assertive when advocating for your needs. Assertive people place their needs on an **equal** level with the needs of others. If you are assertive, you try to find **mutually satisfactory solutions** that don't trample on the needs of others, yet meet your own unique hearing needs. Unfortunately, few hard of hearing people come out of their passive shells and become assertive, yet this is when successful communication takes place.

As an assertive person, you will be open, honest and direct about your needs. You will express freely your legitimate rights without undue stress and without violating the rights of others.

Although few hard of hearing people are naturally assertive about their hearing needs, the good news is that anyone, including you, can learn to be more assertive. Assertive people approach communication problems in an analytical and cooperative way. Thus, you will seek solutions—here's how we could work this out together—rather than getting angry and blaming others (aggressive), or simply sitting there and doing nothing (passive).

As an assertive person, you will readily admit your hearing loss, assume responsibility for the resulting communication difficulties, and suggest ways to mutually solve them. In doing so, you will use all the coping strategies at your disposal including amplification, speechreading and other communication tips. The result is that you will experience improved communication, comfortable relationships and positive feelings of self-worth.

You can choose how you will cope with your hearing loss. You can either sit back, remain passive and take a "poor me" attitude, or you can choose to assert yourself and become the best hard of hearing person you can be. When you choose this path, you will find that although being hard of hearing is still not easy, you will live a full and rewarding life in spite of your hearing loss. Isn't that what you really want?

Chapter 13

Resources

National Organizations

American Academy of Audiology (AAA)

Website contains information for hard of hearing people and a locator to find the audiologist nearest you.

11730 Plaza America Drive, Suite 300
Reston, VA 20190
Phone: 800-222-2336
FAX: 703-790-8631
Email: infoaud@audiology.org
Website: http://www.audiology.org

American Academy of Otolaryngology—Head and Neck Surgery (AAO-HNS)

Website contains information about ear specialists and what they can do for you. It also includes a locator so you can find ENTs and otologists near you.

1650 Diagonal Road
Alexandria, VA 22314-2857
Phone: 703-836-4444
Email: webmaster@entnet.org
Website: http://www.entnet.org

American Speech-Language-Hearing Association (ASHA)

Website contains information for hard of hearing people and a locator to find audiologists near you.

2200 Research Boulevard
Rockville, MD 20850-3289
Phone: 800-638-8255
Email: actioncenter@asha.org
Website: http://www.asha.org

American Tinnitus Association (ATA)

Provides information, referrals and support for people who experience ringing in their ears and other head noises.

Dept. 4049
Washington, DC 20042-4049
Phone: 800-634-8978
Email directory: https://www.ata.org/about-us/leadership
Website: https://www.ata.org

Association of Late Deafened Adults (ALDA)

Provides resources and information, and promotes awareness of the needs of people who have lost most or all their hearing as adults.

ALDA, Inc.
8038 Macintosh Lane, Suite 2
Rockford, IL 61107
Voice: 815-332-1515
Email: info@alda.org
Website: http://www.alda.org

Beyond Hearing

An on-line discussion group exclusively for hearing loss issues. Post your questions, and you will receive replies from knowledgeable people. To subscribe, either send a blank email to Beyond-Hearing-subscribe@yahoogroups.com or go to http://groups.yahoo.com/group/Beyond-Hearing and click on the button "Join This Group!"

Website: http://groups.yahoo.com/group/Beyond-Hearing/

Center for Hearing Loss Help

Provides more than 1,000 easy-to-read informational articles on hearing loss and other ear problems and successful coping strategies. Also carries some of the best books and assistive listening devices (ALDs) on the market to help hard of hearing people. You can also subscribe to their free e-zine "Hearing Loss Help".

1013 Ridgeway Dr.
Lynden, WA 98264
Phone: 360-778-1266
FAX: 360-389-5226
Email: info@hearinglosshelp.com
Website: http://hearinglosshelp.com

Hearing Loss Association of America

National voice of hard of hearing people in the USA. Devoted to the welfare and interests of hard of hearing people. Provides information and advocacy. Local support chapters throughout the country. Locate the chapter nearest you from their website.

7910 Woodmont Avenue, Suite 1200
Bethesda, MD 20814
Phone: Voice: 301-657-2248
FAX: 301-913-9413
Email: info@hearingloss.org
Website: http://www.hearingloss.org

Hyperacusis Network

Support group for people who have a reduced tolerance to sound—hyperacusis and recruitment.

444 Edgewood Drive
Green Bay, WI 54302
Phone: 920-468-4667
FAX: 920-468-0168
Email: earhelp@yahoo.com
Website: http://www.hyperacusis.net

National Institute on Deafness and Other Communication Disorders (NIDCD) Information Clearinghouse

Provides a wealth of on-line information and free publications on various aspects of hearing loss and ear disorders.

31 Center Drive, MSC 2320
Bethesda, MD 20892-2320
Phone: 800-241-1044
TTY: 800-241-1055
Email: nidcdinfo@nidcd.nih.gov
Website: http://www.nidcd.nih.gov

SayWhat Club

An on-line group (email list) of hard of hearing people that provides help, encouragement, support and friendship to each other via email. In addition to the 5 or 6 "family" lists, there is a specialized list of note:

CI: An excellent information and support list for cochlear implant users and prospective users.

To join the SayWhatClub or for more information contact them at:

Email: info@saywhatclub.com
Website: http://www.saywhatclub.com

Vestibular Disorders Association (VEDA)

Provides information and support for people suffering from inner-ear balance disorders, vertigo and related ear problems. They have a lot of information on-line on their web site including an excellent list of support groups in Canada and the USA.

Box 13305
Portland, OR 97213
Phone: 800-837-8428
FAX: 503-229-8064
Website: http://www.vestibular.org

Selected Sources of Assistive Listening Devices

Center for Hearing Loss Help

1013 Ridgeway Dr.
Lynden, WA 98264
Phone: 360-778-1266
FAX: 360-389-5226
Email: info@hearinglosshelp.com
Website: http://hearinglosshelp.com/shop

HARC Mercantile Ltd.

1111 West Centre Street
Portage, MI 49024
Phone: 800-445-9968
Email: info@harc.com
Website: http://www.harcmercantile.com

Harris Communications, Inc.

15155 Technology Drive
Eden Prairie, MN 55344-2277
Phone: 800-825-6758
Email: info@harriscomm.com
Website: http://www.harriscomm.com

HITEC Group

1743 Quincy Avenue, Unit #155
Naperville, IL 60540
Phone: 800-288-8303
Email: info@hitec.com
Website: http://www.hitec.com

LS&S

145 River Rock Drive
Buffalo, NY 14207
Phone: 800-468-4789
Email: info@LSSproducts.com
Website: http://www.LSSproducts.com

Literature Cited

Alpiner, Jerome G. and Patricia A. McCarthy. 1987. Rehabilitative Audiology: Children and Adults. Williams & Wilkins. Baltimore, MD.

Bauman, Neil G. 2016a. Take Control of Your Tinnitus—Here's How. Integrity First Publications, 1013 Ridgeway Dr., Lynden, WA 98264. http://hearinglosshelp.com/shop/category/books/.

Bauman, Neil G. 2016b. Say Good Bye to Meniere's Disease—Here's How to Make Your World Stop Spinning. 4th Edition. Integrity First Publications, 1013 Ridgeway Dr., Lynden, WA 98264. http://hearinglosshelp.com/shop/category/books/.

Bauman, Neil G. 2011a. Grieving for Your Hearing Loss. The Rocky Road from Denial to Acceptance. 3rd Edition. Integrity First Publications, 1013 Ridgeway Dr., Lynden, WA 98264. http://hearinglosshelp.com/shop/category/books/.

Bauman, Neil G. 2011b. Hear! Here! You and Your Hearing Loss/You and Your Hearing Aids. 4th Edition. Integrity First Publications, 1013 Ridgeway Dr., Lynden, WA 98264. http://hearinglosshelp.com/shop/category/books/.

Bauman, Neil G. 2011c. Phantom Voices, Ethereal Music & Other Spooky Sounds. 2nd Edition. Integrity First Publications, 1013 Ridgeway Dr., Lynden, WA 98264. http://hearinglosshelp.com/shop/category/books/.

Bauman, Neil G. 2011d. Supersensitive to Sound? You May Have Hyperacusis. 3rd. Edition. Integrity First Publications. 1013 Ridgeway Dr., Lynden, WA 98264. http://hearinglosshelp.com/shop/category/books/.

Bauman, Neil G. 2011e. When Hearing Loss Ambushes Your Ears. 2nd Edition. Integrity First Publications, 1013 Ridgeway Dr., Lynden, WA 98264. http://hearinglosshelp.com/shop/category/books/.

Bauman, Neil G. 2010a. Ototoxic Drugs Exposed. 3rd Edition. Integrity First Publications, 1013 Ridgeway Dr., Lynden, WA 98264. http://hearinglosshelp.com/shop/category/books/.

Bauman, Neil. 2010b. Talking with Hard of Hearing People—Here's How to Do It Right! 3rd Edition. Integrity First Publications. 1013 Ridgeway Dr., Lynden, WA 98264. http://hearinglosshelp.com/shop/category/books/.

Bauman, Neil G. 2008. Hearing Loss Much More Common Than Previously Thought. http://hearinglosshelp.com/blog/hearing-loss-much-more-common-than-previously-thought/.

Bruce, Leslie. 1991. Intimacy and the Hard of Hearing, Part I. In: Listen. Canadian Hard of Hearing Association, Ottawa, ON. Fall edition.

Causes of Hearing Loss in Adults. 2000. Audionics. http://www.audionicsnyc.com/AdultCause.cfm.

Cochlear Implants and Seniors: When Hearing Aids Aren't Enough. 2003. Hearing Loss Association of America 7910 Woodmont Avenue, Suite 1200, Bethesda, MD 20814.

Desai, Mayur, et. al. March 2001. Trends in Vision and Hearing Among Older Americans. Aging Trends No. 2. Centers for Disease Control and Prevention. National Center for Health Statistics.

Discovering and Understanding Tinnitus. 1997. Tinnitus FAQ. http://www.bixby.org/faq/tinnitus/discover.html.

Dobie, Robert, et al. "Tinnitus, Depression, and Ageing" In: *Geriatric Otorhinolaryngology.*

Facts On Hearing Loss. 2003. Hearing Loss Association of America. Bethesda, MD. http://www.hearingloss.org/html/hearing_loss_fact_sheets.html.

Frequently Asked Questions: General Questions About Tinnitus. 2003. American Tinnitus Association. Portland, Oregon. http://www.ata.org/about_tinnitus/consumer/faq.html.

Frequently Asked Questions: Helen Keller Quotations. 2000. Deaf-related Resources. Library Gallaudet University http://library.gallaudet.edu/dr/faq-helen-keller.html.

Holman, B.J. Feb 21, 2002. Email—personal communication. Similar results were published by Alpiner, Jerome G. and Patricia A. McCarthy. 1987. Rehabilitative Audiology: Children and Adults. Williams & Wilkins. Baltimore, MD. pp. 320-321.

Huning, Debbie. 1992. Living Well with Hearing Loss. John Wiley & Sons, Inc. New York.

Jastreboff. 2000. Tinnitus & Hyperacusis Center. Emory University. Atlanta, Georgia. http://www.tinnitus-pjj.com.

Kisor, Henry. 1990. What's That Pig Outdoors? A Memoir of Deafness. Hill & Wang: A Division of Farrar, Straus & Giroux. New York, NY.

Kochkin, Sergei. 1991. What This Industry Needs Is a Marlboro Man. In: ASHA (American Speech-Language Hearing Association). December.

Lin, Frank, et. al. 2011. Hearing Loss Prevalence and Risk Factors Among Older Adults in the United States. J Gerontol A Biol Sci Med Sci (2011). http://biomedgerontology.oxfordjournals.org/content/early/2011/02/27/gerona.glr002.abstract.

McCall, Rosemary. 1991. Hearing Loss?—A Guide to Self-help. Robert Hale Limited. London.

Staab, Dr. Wayne J. 1991. The Rexton Guide to Better Hearing. 512 East Canterbury Lane, Phoenix, Arizona 85022.

Summary Health Statistics for US. Adults: National Health Interview Survey, 1997. May, 2002. Vital and Health Statistics. Series 10, Number 205. Data from the National Health Interview Survey. Department of Health and Human Services, Centers for Disease Control and Prevention, National Center for Health Statistics.

Wantuch, Liz, Ph.D. 2005. Psycho-Social Impact of Hearing Loss. Address given in San Francisco, November 12, 2005.

Good Books on Hearing Loss

Integrity First Books in the series:

Everything You Wanted to Know About Your Hearing Loss But Were Afraid to Ask (Because You Knew You Wouldn't Hear the Answers Anyway!)

by Neil G. Bauman, Ph.D.

If you have enjoyed this book and would like to learn more about hearing loss and how you can successfully live with it, you may be interested in some helpful books by Dr. Neil. Each book is packed with the things you need to know in order to thrive in spite of your various hearing loss issues. The direct link to the following books is at http://hearinglosshelp.com/shop/category/books/.

Ototoxic Drugs Exposed—The Shocking Truth About Prescription Drugs, Medications, Chemicals and Herbals That Can (and Do) Damage Our Ears ($52.45; eBook $39.95)

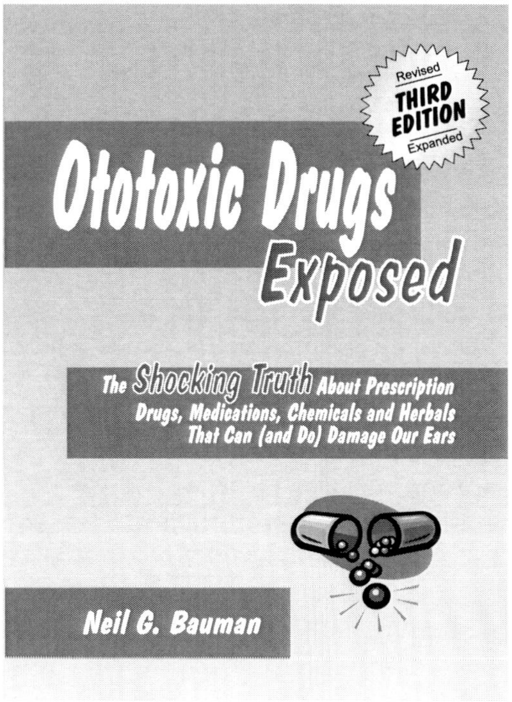

This book, now in its third edition, reveals the shocking truth that many prescription drugs can damage your ears. Some drugs slowly and insidiously rob you of your hearing, cause your ears to ring or destroy your balance. Other drugs can smash your ears in one fell swoop, leaving you with profound, permanent hearing loss and bringing traumatic change into your life. Learn how to protect your ears from the ravages of ototoxic drugs and chemicals. Describes the specific ototoxic effects of 877 drugs, 35 herbals and 148 chemicals (798 pages).

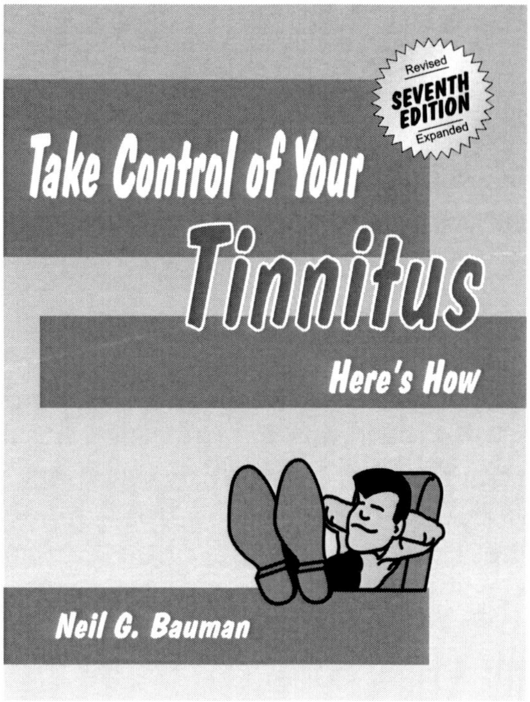

Take Control of Your Tinnitus—Here's How ($29.95; eBook $22.99)

If your ears ring, buzz, chirp, hiss, click or roar, you know just how annoying tinnitus can be. The good news is that you do not have to put up with this racket for the rest of your life. You can take control of your tinnitus. Recent studies show that a lot of what we thought we knew about tinnitus is not true at all. Exciting new research reveals a number of things that you can do to eliminate or greatly reduce the severity of your tinnitus so that it no longer bothers you. This totally-revised, up-to-date and expanded 7th edition contains the very latest in tinnitus research and treatment. In this book you will learn what tinnitus is, what causes tinnitus and things you can do to take control of your tinnitus (356 pages).

Phantom Voices, Ethereal Music & Other Spooky Sounds ($22.49; eBook $16.99)

When you realize you are hearing phantom sounds, you immediately think that something has gone dreadfully wrong "upstairs"—that you are going crazy. Because of this, few people openly talk about the strange phantom voices, music, singing and other spooky sounds they hear. This book, the first of its kind in the world, lifts the veil on "Musical Ear syndrome" and reveals numerous first-hand accounts of the many strange phantom sounds people experience. Not only that, it explains what causes these phantom sounds, and more importantly, what you can do to eliminate them, or at least, bring them under control (178 pages).

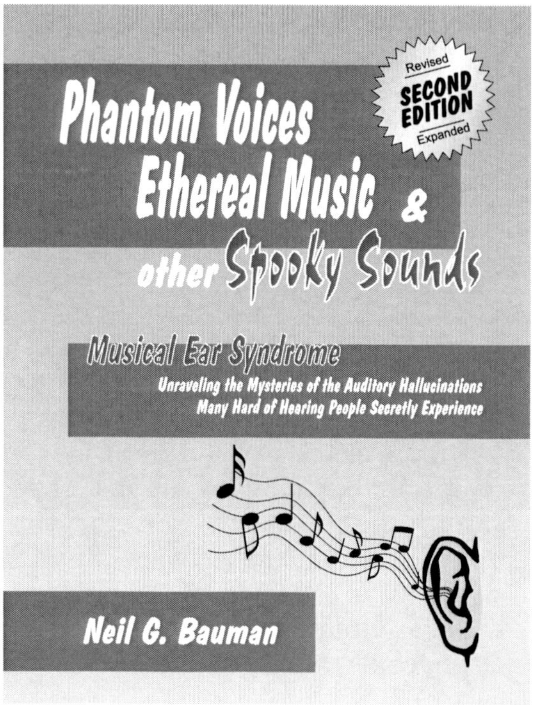

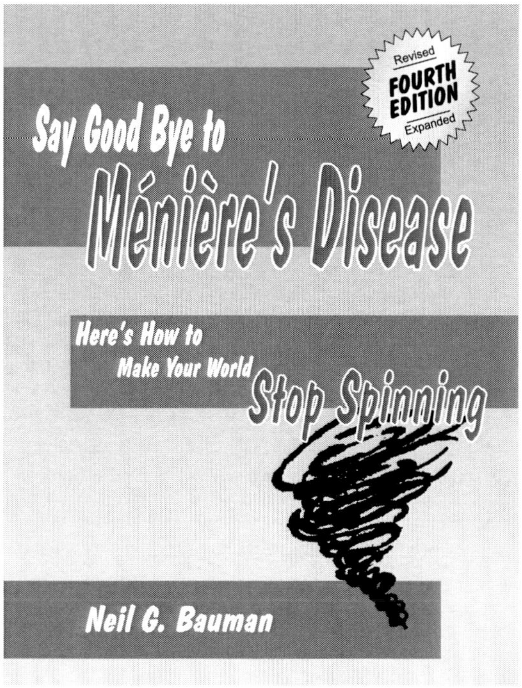

Say Good Bye to Ménière's Disease—Here's How to Make Your World Stop Spinning ($21.95; eBook $16.49)

Ménière's disease is one of the more baffling and incapacitating conditions a person can experience. If you suffer from your world spinning, have a fluctuating hearing loss, tinnitus and a feeling of fullness in your ears, this book is for you. It details what Ménière's disease is like; explains the recent breakthrough into the underlying cause of Ménière's; and shows you how, at last, you can be free from the ravages of this debilitating condition. Each page is packed with practical information to help you successfully conquer your Meniere's disease. Join the hundreds and hundreds of people whose worlds have now stopped spinning (128 pages).

Keys to Successfully Living with Your Hearing Loss ($19.97; eBook $15.49)

Do you know: a) the critical missing element to successfully living with your hearing loss? b) that the No. 1 coping strategy hard of hearing people instinctively use is wrong, wrong, wrong? c) what the single most effective hearing loss coping strategy is? d) how you can turn your hearing aids into awesome hearing devices? This book addresses the surprising answers to these and other critical questions. Applying them to your life will put you well on the road to successfully living with your hearing loss (84 pages).

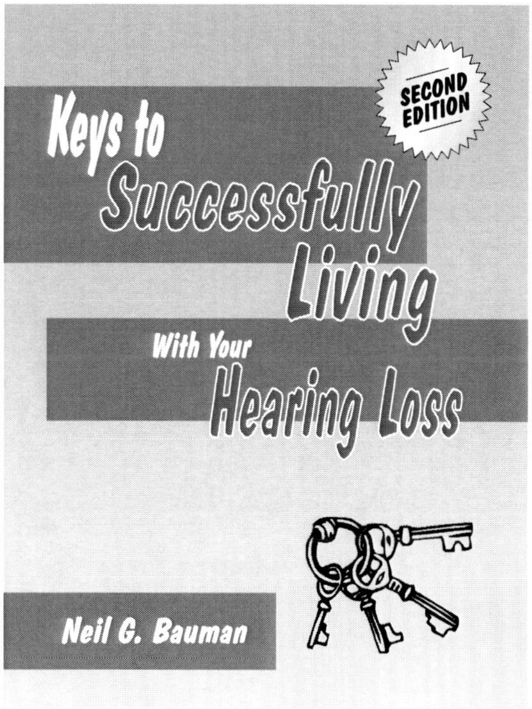

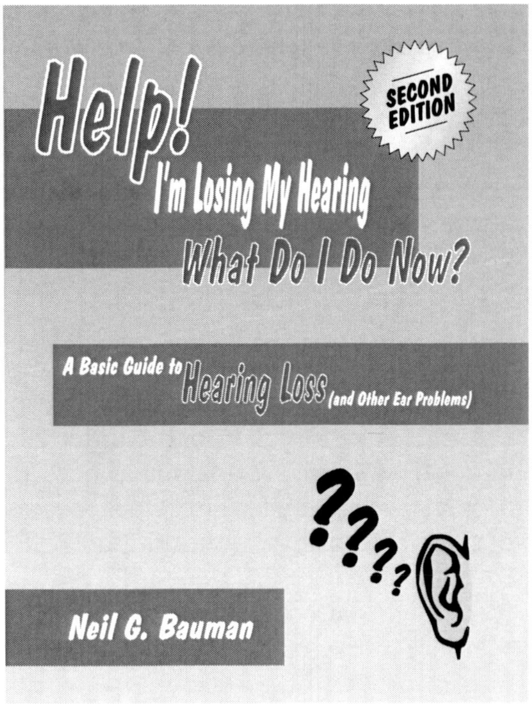

Help! I'm Losing My Hearing—What Do I Do Now? ($18.95; eBook $14.49)

Losing your hearing can flip your world upside down and leave your mind in a turmoil. You may be full of fears, wondering how you will be able to live the rest of your life as a hard of hearing person. You don't know where to turn. You lament, "What do I do now?" Set your mind at rest. This easy to read book, written by a fellow hard of hearing person, is packed with the information and resources you need to successfully deal with your hearing loss and other ear conditions (116 pages).

Grieving for Your Hearing Loss—The Rocky Road from Denial to Acceptance ($12.95; eBook $9.95)

When you lose your hearing you need to grieve. This is not optional—but critical to your continued mental and physical health. This book leads you through the process of dealing with the grief and pain you experience as a result of your hearing loss. It explains what you are going through each step of the way. It gives you hope when you are in the depths of despair and depression. It shows you how you can lead a happy vibrant life again in spite of your hearing loss. This book has helped many (56 pages).

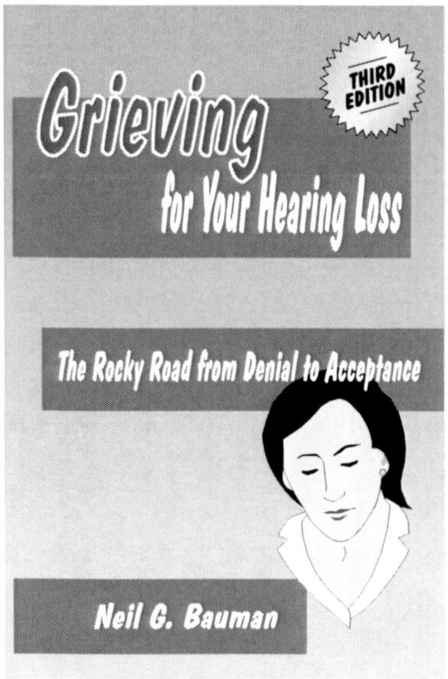

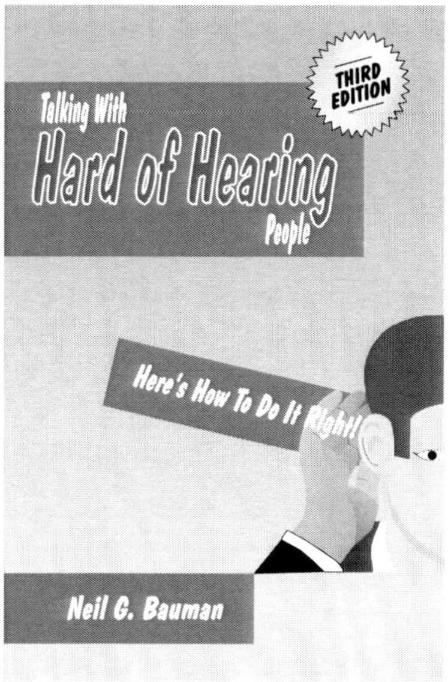

Talking with Hard of Hearing People—Here's How to Do It Right! ($9.95; eBook $7.95)

Talking is important to all of us. When communication breaks down, we all suffer. For hard of hearing people this happens all the time. This book is for you—whether you are hearing or hard of hearing! It explains how to communicate with hard of hearing people in one-to-one situations, in groups and meetings, in emergency situations, and in hospitals and nursing homes. When you use the principles given in this book, good things will happen and you will finally be able to have a comfortable chat with a hard of hearing person (38 pages).

When Hearing Loss Ambushes Your Ears—Here's What Happens When Your Hearing Goes on the Fritz ($14.95; eBook $11.95)

Hearing loss often blind-sides you. As a result, your first step should be to learn as much as you can about your hearing loss; then you will be able to cope better. This most interesting book explains how your ears work, the causes of hearing loss, what you can expect to hear with different levels of hearing loss and why you often can't understand what you hear. Lots of audiograms and charts help make things clear. You will also discover a lot of fascinating things about how loud noises damage your ears (88 pages).

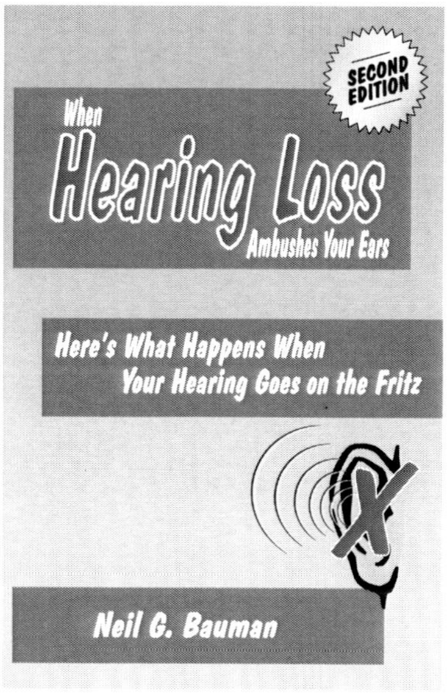

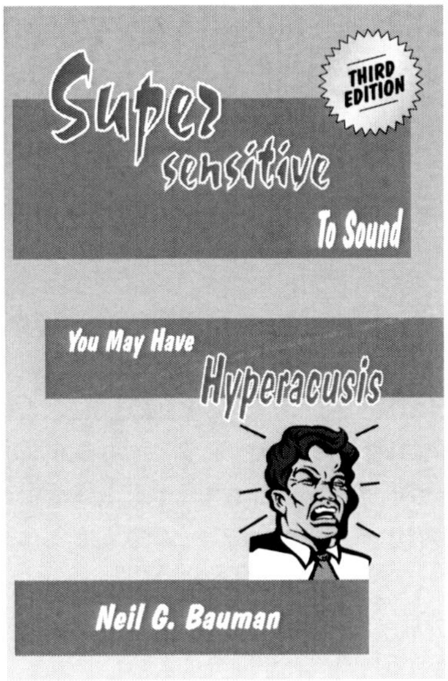

Supersensitive to Sound? You May Have Hyperacusis ($9.95; eBook $7.95)

If some (or all) normal sounds seem so loud they blow your socks off, this is the book you want to read! You don't have to avoid noise or lock yourself away in a soundproof room. Exciting new research on this previously baffling problem reveals what you can do to help bring your hyperacusis under control (42 pages).

Hear! Here! You and Your Hearing Loss/You and Your Hearing Aids ($12.95; eBook $10.95)

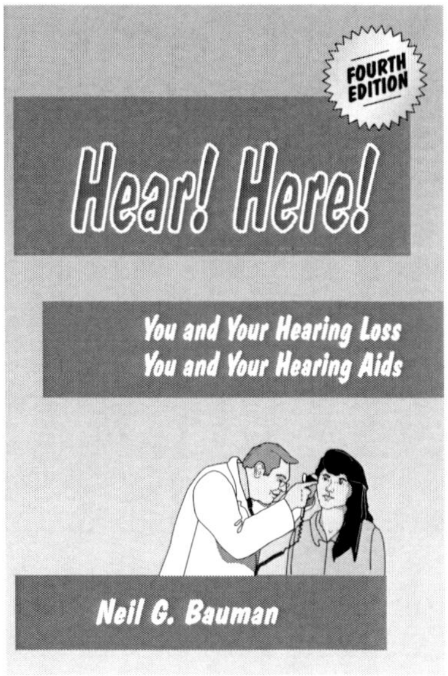

Part I of this book contains a series of my newspaper articles on hearing loss such as, "Hear Today. Gone Tomorrow?" "Hearing Loss Is Sneaky!" "The Wages of Din Is Deaf!" "When Your Ears Ring..." "Get In My Face Before You Speak!" "How's That Again?" "Being Hard of Hearing Is Hard" "I'm Deaf, Not Daft!" Part II contains articles on hearing aids such as, "You Better Watch Out..." "Before Buying Your First Hearing Aid..." "Please Don't Lock Me Away in Your Drawer" "Good-bye World of Silence!" "Becoming Friends with Your Hearing Aids" "Two's Better Than One!" (56 pages).

You can order any of the foregoing books/eBooks (plus you can read more than 1,000 other helpful articles about hearing loss and related issues) from the

Center for Hearing Loss Help

web site at

http://hearinglosshelp.com

or order them from the address below

Center for Hearing Loss Help

1013 Ridgeway Drive,
Lynden, WA 98264-1057
Phone: (360) 778-1266
FAX: (360) 389-5226
E-mail: info@hearinglosshelp.com
Web site: http://hearinglosshelp.com

Made in United States
North Haven, CT
29 November 2025

83237203R00065